AF557805

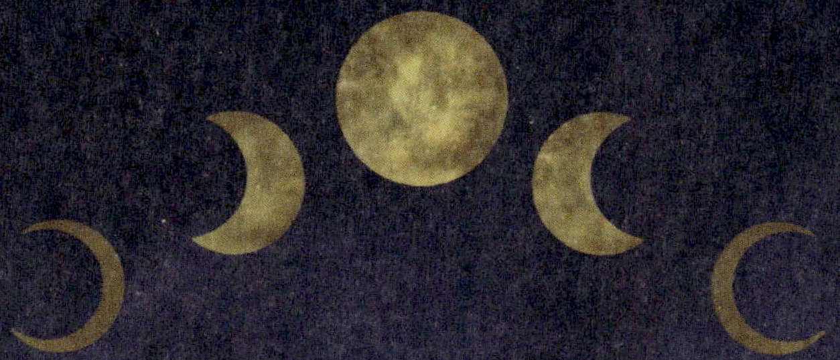

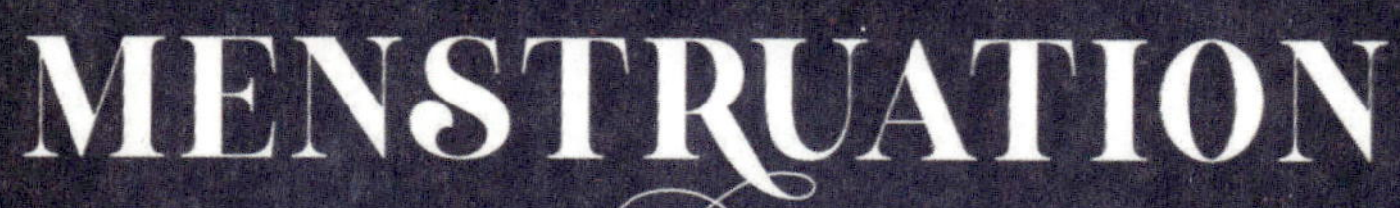

MENSTRUATION

Moon, Men and More

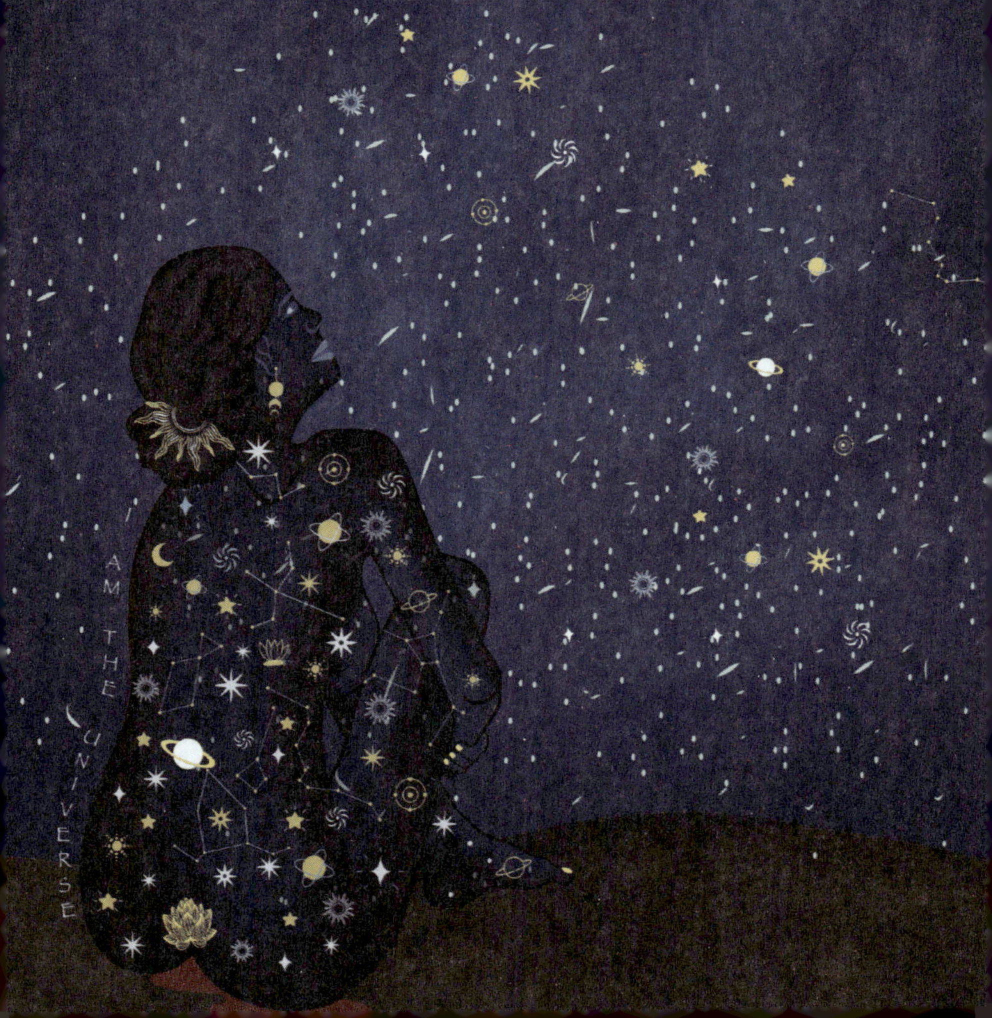

MENSTRUATION

Moon, Men and More

NIRMALA GOWDA NAYAK

Illustrations by Sarah Mae Quezon

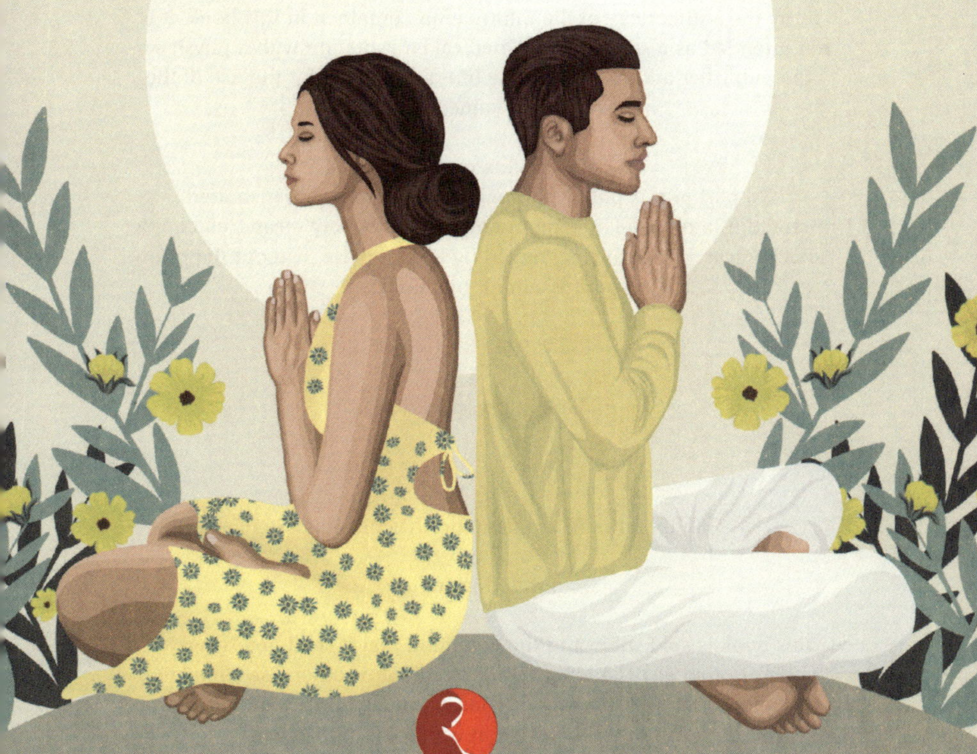

RUPA

Published by
Rupa Publications India Pvt. Ltd 2024
7/16, Ansari Road, Daryaganj
New Delhi 110002

Sales centres:
Bengaluru Chennai
Hyderabad Jaipur Kathmandu
Kolkata Mumbai Prayagraj

Illustrations by Sarah Mae Quezon

P-ISBN: 978-93-6156-596-0

First impression 2024

10 9 8 7 6 5 4 3 2 1

Printed in India

Dedicated to every woman,
in celebration of our shared journey.

ꕥ

CONTENTS

INTRODUCTION

'Women are glorified for being fertile,
while ostracized for the blood that makes them so.'

—RAJVI DESAI

Across numerous cultures and traditions, the womb has been deeply revered as a source of sacred energy and fertility and acknowledged as the wellspring of life. The Kamakhya Temple in India (one of the oldest 4 of the 51 *shakti peethas* located on the Nilachal Hills in Assam) celebrates its menstruating goddess by worshipping the aniconic *yoni* (or womb) and conducts the Ambubachi Mela, which marks the yearly menstruation course of goddess Kamakhya.

As patriarchy became all-pervasive, the womb's significance diminished, relegating it to a mere reproductive organ rather than celebrating it as a symbol of female strength and power. Women have endured a history of negative connotations and stigmas surrounding menstruation, and their reproductive health has never been prioritized. Even today, menstruation remains a taboo topic in many parts of the world, consequently affecting women's well-being, mindset, lifestyle and, most importantly, health. It is imperative that we rediscover the womb's magnificence, and recognize its pivotal role in our lives as the cradle of human existence and a symbol of feminine power.

It is time to rekindle our appreciation for the true splendour of the womb and celebrate and honour this extraordinary part of the female anatomy. Women should take pride in their innate power to bring forth new life into the world. It is time to break free from the negative societal attitudes that have tarnished the natural process of menstruation and reclaim power over our own bodies.

MODERN CHALLENGES

In the modern world, women are often conditioned to perceive menstruation, an inseparable aspect of their nature, as a hindrance to societal progress. They are expected to juggle daily responsibilities, jobs and chores at the cost of their personal growth and well-being. The high-stress lifestyle and demands of a competitive, tech-driven world has created self-imposed pressures, leading many women to disconnect from their true nature (*prakriti*). This alienation can lead to emotional and physical discomfort, affecting both body and mind.

Women menstruate because they are 'humans with wombs'. In these times, it is more important than ever to approach this natural occurrence holistically. To embrace womanhood is to understand the sacredness of the bleeding phase and comprehend the magic and rhythm of nature and the Moon.

INCLUSIVENESS

I firmly believe that the journey of menstrual awareness should no longer be confined to women alone. It is equally about engaging men from all walks of life who play vital roles in women's lives as fathers, spouses, brothers, partners, friends and sons. They must be educated, included and made aware that their existence is intricately connected to the physical process of menstruation. This revelation aims to dismantle the conditioned perceptions of women and their roles in today's world.

Consequently, awareness programs should commence at primary levels, educating both boys and girls about the menstrual process, hormonal variations and the importance of using appropriate anatomical terms when discussing reproductive organs. Promoting inclusivity and understanding from an early age can cultivate a society that recognizes menstrual health, reduces stigma and fosters respect across all genders.

It is imperative that men respect and acknowledge a woman's role to be as significant as a man's in coexistence and cooperation. We need to make a conscious choice to actively include men in the conversation.

SHIFTING MINDSETS

Nearly half the world's population consists of men, and the majority of them have limited knowledge about menstruation. The other half of the population, comprising women, may be unaware to some extent about many aspects of menstruation due to societal stigmas and the absence of open dialogue on the subject.

My aim here is to shift the mindset of both genders and foster a deep understanding of menstruation. Men should step forward, acknowledge and support women by helping eradicate the stigma and taboos that surround the female body. Similarly, women are encouraged to empower themselves, share their experiences and contribute to dismantling these stigmas. By fostering open discussion, we can create a supportive environment that respects and understands menstruation, benefitting society as a whole.

ADDRESSING ALL CONCERNS

To the wonderful women reading this, whether you seek a better understanding of your cycle or effective ways to manage its manifestations, *Menstruation: Moon, Men and More* aims to be a comprehensive resource. It not only offers extensive references but also serves as a practical guide. Within its pages lie invaluable information, designed to promote comprehension, acceptance and mastery over menstrual challenges. It is a guide for anyone wishing to learn more about period blood and revitalize their well-being.

By embracing a natural and holistic approach, this book covers a spectrum of health concerns relevant to women across all stages of life—from the formative years of adolescence to the wisdom of maturity. It offers fundamental insights into the intricacies of individual body types, nutritional requirements and mindful activities aimed at enhancing feminine energy. Additionally, it delves into the emotional well-being associated with various phases of the menstrual cycle, offering guidance to women for navigating their unique paths with resilience, grace and an understanding of their bodies, fostering a lifelong journey of well-being and self-fulfilment.

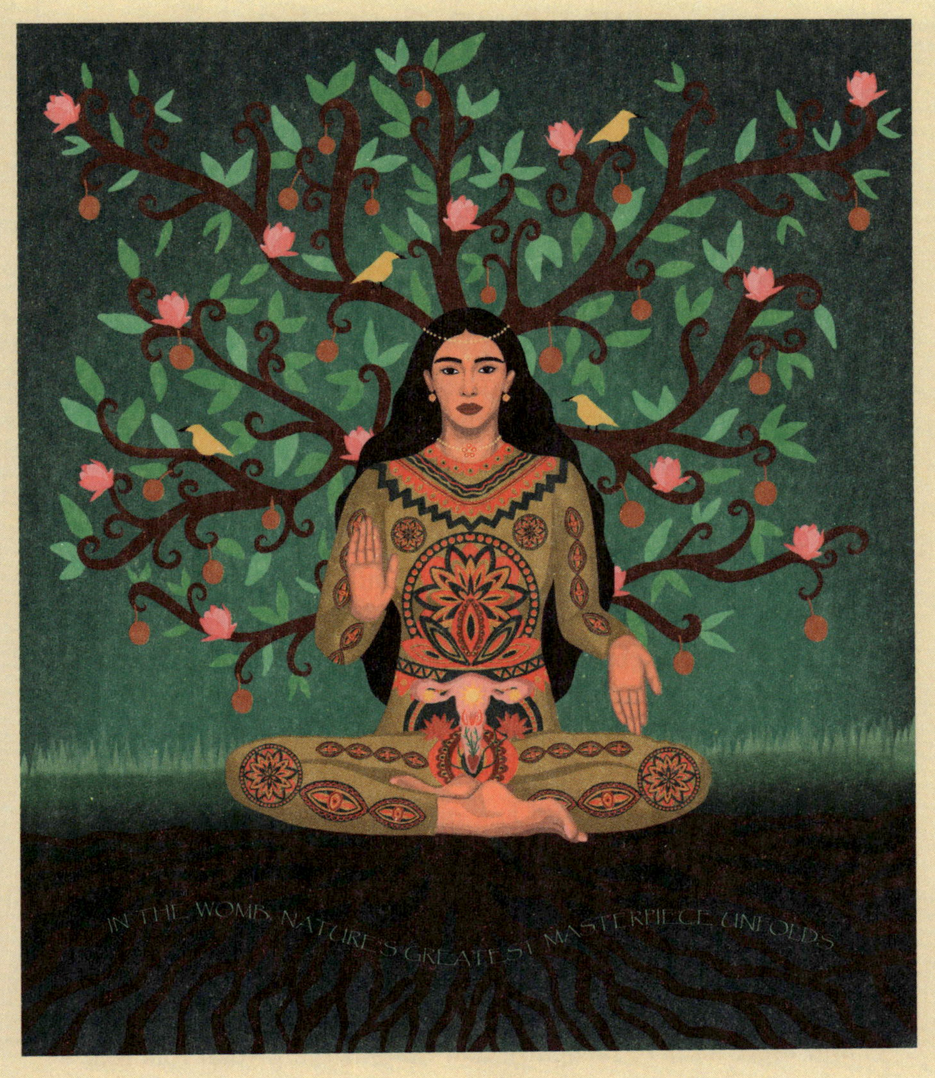
IN THE WOMB, NATURE'S GREATEST MASTERPIECE UNFOLDS

1

THE FOUR PHASES

'The womb of a woman is the gateway to the Universe.'

—ANONYMOUS

A woman is truly a magnificent creation, her crown of magnificence bestowed primarily because of the amazing organ she is born with—the womb.

For millennia, humanity has revered the womb of the divine mother as the origin of human life and creation. The inner light it emanates remains untainted, a radiant force only amplified by her extraordinary capacity to usher life into existence.

The female reproductive system, which encompasses the menstrual cycle, is intricately designed to prepare women for motherhood and progeny. You might find yourself contemplating what makes this aspect of a woman's body so remarkable and why it is a revered subject in our ancient scriptures.[1] Could it be because of its remarkable ability to create, nurture and safeguard life?

My intention with this book is to empower women by nurturing an understanding and fostering appreciation for the versatile guardian of the womb. *Menstruation: Moon, Men and More* aims to recognize and honour the pivotal role that

[1]'Garbha Upanishad: Conception and Growth of a Child in Mother's Womb', *Sanskriti Magazine*, https://www.sanskritimagazine.com/garbha-upanishad-conception-growth-child-mothers-womb/.

the reproductive system plays in a woman's life, serving as a wellspring of creation, intuition and boundless potential.

THE FEMALE REPRODUCTIVE SYSTEM

First, let us delve into the anatomy of the female reproductive system and gain a deeper understanding of its basic functions. Following that we will also explore the intricacies of the menstrual cycle and the nuances of the uterus.

A woman's reproductive system includes a multitude of vital organs that collaborate to facilitate reproduction, pregnancy, fertility and childbirth. Beyond these fundamental roles, it serves as the primary source of female sex hormones, notably, oestrogen and progesterone. These hormones play pivotal roles in regulating the menstrual cycle, supporting embryo implantation and sustaining a healthy pregnancy. In addition to their reproductive functions, oestrogen and progesterone also exert influence over various aspects of a woman's overall health.[2]

The womb undergoes a unique and unparalleled phenomenon called menstruation. I call it 'unique' because no other process can boast of such mind-boggling and exceptional activities that help in creating life.

Let's explore the individual parts of the female reproductive system in detail.[3]

Uterus: The uterus, also referred to as the womb, is a vital reproductive organ in a female's body. It is an inverted, pear-

[2]Cirino, Erica, 'Estrogen vs. Progesterone: Functions in the Human Body,' *Healthline*, Healthline Media, 26 July 2022, https://www.healthline.com/health/womens-health/estrogen-vs-progesterone.

[3]'Female Reproductive System,' *Cleveland Clinic*, 28 November 2022, https://my.clevelandclinic.org/health/articles/9118-female-reproductive-system.

shaped, muscular organ that measures about 6–8 cm in length and is located between the bladder and the rectum. The uterus has four major regions: the fundus (broad, curved upper area where fallopian tubes connect to the uterus), the corpus (main body below the fallopian tubes), the isthmus (lower, narrow neck of the main body) and the cervix (lowest section of the isthmus that opens into the vagina).[4]

The uterus is designed to not just accommodate a growing foetus but is also capable of stretching to aid the latter's growth. It houses the ovaries, fallopian tubes and vagina, and plays a crucial role in the menstrual cycle, fertilization, pregnancy and childbirth.

Ovaries: These are small, oval-shaped glands located on either side of the uterus. Ovaries help in producing and releasing oocytes (eggs). They secrete oestrogen and progesterone, which are vital for controlling the menstrual cycle and pregnancy.

Fallopian tubes: These are a pair of hollow, narrow tubes that link the ovaries to either side of the womb and are lined with hair-like extensions, which help transport the oocyte from the ovaries to the uterus. Also known as uterine tubes, they are considered to be the site of fertilization. Once the fertilized egg travels down this tube and gets embedded in the uterus, the growth of the embryo is set in motion.

Vagina: Also known as the birth canal, the vagina is an elastic, muscular canal lined with nerves and mucous membranes. It connects the uterus and the cervix to the outside of the body. The vaginal opening allows menstrual blood to exit your body. Menstrual cups and tampons are inserted into the vagina through the vaginal opening.

[4]'Uterus,' *Encyclopedia Britannica*, 5 September 2023, https://www.britannica.com/science/uterus.

The uterus, along with the cervix, plays a pivotal role in contributing to the sensations experienced during sexual climax. The network of blood vessels and nerves within the uterus directs blood flow to the pelvis and the external genitalia, including the vagina, labia and clitoris for sexual response. The uterus also provides structural integrity and support to the bladder, bowel, pelvic bones and other organs. During childbirth, the uterus creates rhythmic contractions to help in the smooth delivery of the baby.

Cervix: The cervix, a crucial component of the female reproductive system, serves as the gateway between the uterus and the vagina. Remarkably adaptable, it transforms during the menstrual cycle, thickening to safeguard the uterus during non-fertile periods and softening to facilitate the passage of sperm during ovulation. During childbirth, the cervix plays a monumental role by dilating to allow the baby's passage. Beyond its mechanical functions, the cervix also secretes mucus, contributing to fertility by creating a conducive environment for sperm transport. This multifaceted organ stands as a testament to the intricate orchestration of the female reproductive system, harmonizing its functions to support the continuum of life.

Menstruation transcends mere biological processes, and encompasses profound wisdom, which needs to be grasped before assessing whether the stigma surrounding menstruation is warranted.

THE GREAT MENSTRUAL CYCLE

The term 'great' is the crown I have given to menstruation for all the goodness it bestows on a woman, particularly to those who are attuned to its astounding powers.

The monthly occurrence of a woman's menstrual cycle has

been divided into four phases based on hormonal variations.[5] The menstrual cycle is a biofeedback system as each phase is interdependent on the functioning of other phases.[6] The four distinct phases of the menstrual cycle are the menstrual, follicular, ovulatory and luteal phases.

The menstrual phase marks the beginning of the menstrual cycle, typically lasting around 3–7 days. It begins with the shedding of the uterine lining (endometrium) that has built up in the previous cycle as a result of decreased levels of oestrogen and progesterone. This shedding leads to menstrual bleeding, commonly known as a woman's period. The menstrual phase initiates the reproductive cycle, preparing the uterus for a potential pregnancy in the subsequent phases.

In the follicular phase, the pituitary gland releases follicle-stimulating hormone (FSH), stimulating the growth of ovarian follicles. This surge in oestrogen readies the uterus for potential implantation.

The ovulatory phase marks the pinnacle of the cycle, triggered by a surge in luteinizing hormone (LH), causing the mature follicle to release an egg.

The luteal phase is characterized by the ruptured follicle transforming into the corpus luteum, which secretes progesterone to prepare the uterus for a potential embryo. If fertilization doesn't occur, hormone levels decline, initiating the menstrual phase anew. Let us now discuss these phases in detail.

[5]Watson, Stephanie, 'Stages of the Menstrual Cycle', *Healthline*, Healthline Media, 13 March 2023, https://www.healthline.com/health/womens-health/stages-of-menstrual-cycle.

[6]'The Menstrual (Period) Cycle,' *Sexual Health Victoria*, https://shvic.org.au/for-you/reproductive-and-sexual-health/menstrual-cycle.

Menstrual Phase

Menstruation, a vital aspect of a woman's monthly cycle, is the process through which the uterine lining is shed, resulting in the discharge of blood and other materials through the vagina. This natural occurrence typically lasts from 3 to 7 days and repeats approximately every 25–35 days from puberty till menopause.

During the phases of the menstrual cycle, the uterus undergoes intricate changes to receive a fertilized egg for a potential pregnancy. If fertilization does not occur, the thickened endometrial lining of the uterus is shed, leading to the expulsion of menstrual blood every month. This cycle is regulated by the hypothalamus, a deep-seated part of the brain that controls the endocrine hormones and influences the pituitary gland. The pituitary is the master gland affecting various aspects of a woman's metabolism, sex drive and menstrual cycle.

The entire menstrual cycle is measured from the first day of bleeding to the commencement of the next period. Although it is normal to have a shorter or longer monthly cycle, for most women, the average length of a period can range between 1 day and 7 days. It is normal for women to lose about 4–5 tablespoons (30–80 ml) of blood over the span of three days.

The blood's colour can range from deep reds and browns to pink. The deeper hues indicate that the blood has taken a bit longer to leave the uterus and has oxidized, and if the colour is hibiscus red, it indicates that the blood is fresh, without any odour.[7]

This natural elimination of menstrual blood prepares the body for a new cycle of ovulation. This monthly occurrence can be predicted by keeping track of the cyclical pattern in a journal.

---

[7]Eske, Jamie, 'What Does the Color of Period Blood Mean?', *Medical News Today*, Healthline Media, 23 November 2023, https://www.medicalnewstoday.com/articles/324848.

The strong contractions of the uterus that aid the shedding of the uterine lining can lead to a woman experiencing uncomfortable symptoms, such as cramps, bloating and lower back pain. Severe and painful contractions are not normal and are triggered by prostaglandins,[8] a natural chemical produced in the body. Excess prostaglandins produced in the body can result in painful contractions. Women must be cautious of consuming excess oestrogen-rich foods (detailed in Chapter 10) that are more likely to thicken the uterine lining, thus creating more prostaglandins, leading to severe pain during the bleeding period. These contractions can also momentarily constrict the blood vessels throughout the body, leading to fatigue and mood fluctuations.[9]

Based on the hormonal riot occurring during this phase, experts have compared the bleeding process to a miniature prenatal, and have stressed the importance of nourishing the body with food and care. Symbolically, a bleeding vagina is also considered a 'weeping womb' as pregnancy could not take place like the body anticipated, which prompts the uterus to undergo a process of recovery.[10]

Menstruation isn't just a women's issue. It's a human issue. Thus, there is a greater need for all individuals, including men, to cultivate compassion and educate themselves about the menstrual cycle and the chemistry of period blood. Accurate knowledge is crucial in dispelling unwarranted fallacies around menstrual blood.

---

[8]Hersh, Erica, 'Why Do I Feel Light-Headed During My Period?,' *Healthline*, Healthline Media, 9 August 2019, https://www.healthline.com/health/womens-health/dizziness-before-period.

[9]Walters, Meg, 'How to Work with Your Period, Not Against It,' *Healthline*, Healthline Media, 26 August 2020, https://www.healthline.com/health/make-your-period-work-for-you.

[10]Yager, Sarah, 'Weeping of a Disappointed Womb,' *The Atlantic*, The Atlantic Monthly Group, 2 October 2013, https://www.theatlantic.com/health/archive/2013/10/weeping-of-a-disappointed-womb/280166/.

The Essence of Menstrual Blood

The menstrual blood is enriched with essential nutrients. It consists of broken-down endometrial tissue, blood from the uterine arteries, cervical mucus and unfertilized eggs from the previous cycle. The decrease in oestrogen and progesterone levels triggers the shedding of the endometrium, which is enriched with blood from the two uterine arteries, providing nourishment to the embryo and serving as the initial source of blood from the mother to the baby.

The common misconception about period blood is that it is impure and repulsive. However, components of the expelled endometrial fluid have traces of iron, potassium, sodium chloride, water and glucose and are also rich in menstrual blood-derived stem/stromal cells (MenSCs).[11] During menstruation, women create abundant, free sources of stem cells every month and research has proven that there are ways to successfully and non-invasively use them in treating various ailments.[12]

Menstruation and menstrual blood are crucial aspects of human biology, contributing to our existence and vitality.

It is essential for all genders to reflect upon this revelation and give menstruation and menstrual blood the dignity and respect they deserve.

Follicular Phase

The follicular phase revolves around the maturation of the egg inside the ovaries. This phase is considered the longest phase,

[11] Motluck, Alison, 'Menstrual Blood Could Be Rich Source of Stem Cells,' *NewScientist*, 15 November 2007, https://www.newscientist.com/article/dn12924-menstrual-blood-could-be-rich-source-of-stem-cells/.

[12] Chen, Lijun, Jingjing Qu, Tianli Cheng, Xin Chen, and Charlie Xiang, 'Menstrual Blood-derived Stem Cells: Toward Therapeutic Mechanisms, Novel Strategies, and Future Perspectives in the Treatment of Diseases,' *Stem Cell Research & Therapy*, Vol. 10, No. 1, 2019, 406, https://doi.org/10.1186/s13287-019-1503-7.

which begins on the first day of menstruation and continues until ovulation. This typically spans from 14 to 21 days. There are a lot of activities that happen in and around the ovaries during this phase, accompanied by an increase in the production of oestrogen in the body. The surge in hormones triggers the hypothalamus in the brain, which in turn signals the pituitary gland to release FSH.[13] The FSH then prepares the uterus for pregnancy by stimulating the ovaries to produce around 5–20 tiny sacs called follicles that bead on its surface. Each follicle contains an egg waiting to mature.

These maturing follicles stimulate the uterus to thicken its walls and create a nutrient-rich environment in preparation for a possible pregnancy. Eventually, only one follicle matures into an egg. This phase, which normally occurs on day 10 of the 28-day menstrual cycle, can signal a surge of hormones within the body. While this hormonal upsurge makes some women feel confident and they radiate energy, it can also induce low energy and mood swings in individuals with hormone imbalances.

Ovulatory Phase

Ovulation refers to the release of a mature egg from one of the ovaries, occurring approximately from day 14 to day 17 in a menstrual cycle. The oestrogen levels, which were low at the beginning of the menstrual cycle, keep rising to signal the ovaries to release the egg.

This is the period when one dominant and mature egg outshines all other follicles in the ovary and travels down the fallopian tube towards the uterus, where it gets fertilized by the sperm; if it doesn't fuse with the sperm within this duration, it dies.

---

[13]'Follicle-Stimulating Hormone (FSH)', *Cleveland Clinic*, 23 January 2023, https://my.clevelandclinic.org/health/articles/24638-follicle-stimulating-hormone-fsh.

A woman normally ovulates on the 14th day of an average 28-day menstrual cycle. However, this timing can vary each month for every woman. The period for conception lasts for approximately 24 hours, during which both oestrogen and progesterone levels peak, facilitating the chances of conception.

The hypothalamus in the brain recognizes these rising levels and releases a chemical called gonadotropin.[14] This hormone triggers the pituitary gland to release LH and FSH, making this the best time to conceive. Clear, wet, vaginal secretions and a slight increase in basal body temperature are indications that the womb is ready for conception. The surge in LH levels can be detected in urine and measured with the help of over-the-counter ovulation kits to help a woman detect when she is ovulating.[15]

Luteal Phase

The luteal phase begins in the second half of your cycle, after the ovulation period is over, and ends when your next period starts. This can last from day 14 to day 28 of a menstrual cycle. This is the stage that brings about a transformation in the follicles once the egg is released from the ovary. The ruptured follicles are then transformed into a structure known as the corpus luteum, which starts releasing progesterone, along with a small amount of oestrogen, in anticipation of pregnancy.

This phase is further subdivided based on whether ovulation has occurred in the previous phase or not. If the egg has been fertilized, the uterus prepares itself for the egg to be implanted in the lining of the uterus. The hormone

---

[14]'Gonadotropin-releasing Hormone (GnRH)', *Cleveland Clinic,* 18 March 2022, https://my.clevelandclinic.org/health/body/22525-gonadotropin-releasing-hormone.

[15]'Ovulation', *Cleveland Clinic,* 8 July 2022, https://my.clevelandclinic.org/health/articles/23439-ovulation.

called human chorionic gonadotropin (hCG) is then produced to maintain the functioning of the corpus luteum. The same hormone, when detected in a urine test, confirms pregnancy.[16]

However, if the egg has not been fertilized, the corpus luteum starts to break down within 9–11 days after the ovulation period, leading to a fall in progesterone and oestrogen levels. The rise and fall in progesterone towards the end of the menstrual cycle causes mood swings, food cravings, bloating, weight gain, changes in sexual desire and migraines, which require care and consideration as the body's immunity levels are also low during this period. These emotional and physical upheavals are commonly known as premenstrual syndrome (PMS), which manifests before the onset of the period. The sudden drop in oestrogen and progesterone levels causes the first bleeding phase—repeating the menstrual cycle all over again.

Ensuring healthy progesterone levels is crucial, particularly if there's no plan for conception, as this hormone significantly influences mood regulation by improving sleep quality. Hence, it is recommended to prioritize rest, such as sleeping an extra hour or two if you are feeling fatigued, to help maintain energy levels.

THE WOMB—A FORGOTTEN ENERGY CENTRE

'The womb has a consciousness of its own.'

—MELANIE SWAN

The womb should not merely be regarded as an anatomical structure; instead, it should be viewed and recognized as one of the most powerful energy centres in a woman's body. The

[16]'Human Chorionic Gonadotropin,' *Cleveland Clinic*, 11 November 2022, https://my.clevelandclinic.org/health/articles/22489-human-chorionic-gonadotropin.

entire human race continues to thrive today because of this dynamic, persuasive and spirited hub, which is vital for creating and nurturing life.

Society has certainly played its part by shifting priorities, adding tenacious biological taboos and attaching stigmas to the menstrual phenomenon, resulting in an indifferent attitude towards menstruation. Additionally, prioritizing external and materialistic goals has diverted focus from necessary self-care, causing emotional and physical imbalance.

For a long time, people have been misinformed about the menstrual cycle due to flawed and misguided beliefs. Hence, young women must strive to unlearn and overcome a long history of societal shame and embrace the importance of menstrual health. It is time for us to realize its significance and treat menstruation as a blessing from nature.

The Miracle

The uterus is a strong, super stretchy organ that houses one of the strongest muscles in the body. This wondrous organ can change itself from the size of a pear to a huge balloon, expanding to nearly 20 times its normal size during pregnancy to house a foetus. After delivery, it reverts to its original size. No other organ is as versatile nor can it grow another human life, thus making it worthy of being called the 'miracle organ.'

The Magical

Indian mythology states that the entire universe could be seen inside Lord Krishna's mouth. If truth be told, one would be astonished to know that the entire universe is also contained inside the womb. The womb is the creative centre of existence in the universe and is not only strongly connected to wisdom but also connected to the astronomical cycles of the Earth, Sun and Moon. Isn't it magical to be able to manifest the life one wants to enjoy and also be able to pass on the same legacy to the next generation?

The Mystical

Scientists have made great progress in understanding the female reproductive system but the womb still holds an aura of mystery. Studies have confirmed that a female foetus is born with all the eggs she will ever need in her lifetime.[17] They exist in her ovaries even when she is a 4-month-old foetus. The cellular life of an egg thus begins in one's grandmother's womb. Isn't it astounding that we are connected to our mother and grandmother as a tiny egg in our mother's ovary even before she was born, and when our grandmother was carrying our mother in her womb.[18] Isn't this nature's unparalleled mystery?

> *'If the cardiologist thinks the heart is a wonderful organ, the cardiologist has never heard of the uterus.'*
>
> —ELMAR P. SAKALA

Indeed, it is time to honour and celebrate this wondrous and mystical organ by maintaining its health. Activating our womb energy can guide us towards new dimensions of life, which can be the only way to reclaim the divine power bestowed upon us.

THE BOTTOM LINE

The womb symbolizes the dual nature of life—a nexus of birth and death. Ancient Hindu philosophy keenly acknowledges this

[17]Lewis, Rhona, 'How Many Eggs Are Women Born With? And Other Questions About Egg Supply', *Healthline*, Healthline Media, 4 May 2023, https://www.healthline.com/health/womens-health/how-many-eggs-does-a-woman-have.
[18]Kardia, Sharon, and Tevah Platt, 'In Your Grandmother's Womb: The Egg That Made You', *Gene Doe*, 29 September 2010, https://genedoe.wordpress.com/2010/09/29/in-your-grandmothers-womb-the-egg-that-made-you/.

paradox, illustrating how it serves as a canvas where a new life awaits creation while also shedding the vestiges of old blood and past experiences.

It propagates the wisdom that death is merely a transition—a gateway to a stronger and improved existence. Nature, in its cyclical rhythms, notably through menstruation, serves as a poignant reminder that we possess the innate capacity to release the past and liberate ourselves from the shackles of painful experiences. In doing so, we arise from the ashes like a phoenix repeatedly.

NIMMI'S MANTRA

You are a woman with a womb, creating new life. Move forward fearlessly and seize new opportunities with confidence and bravery.

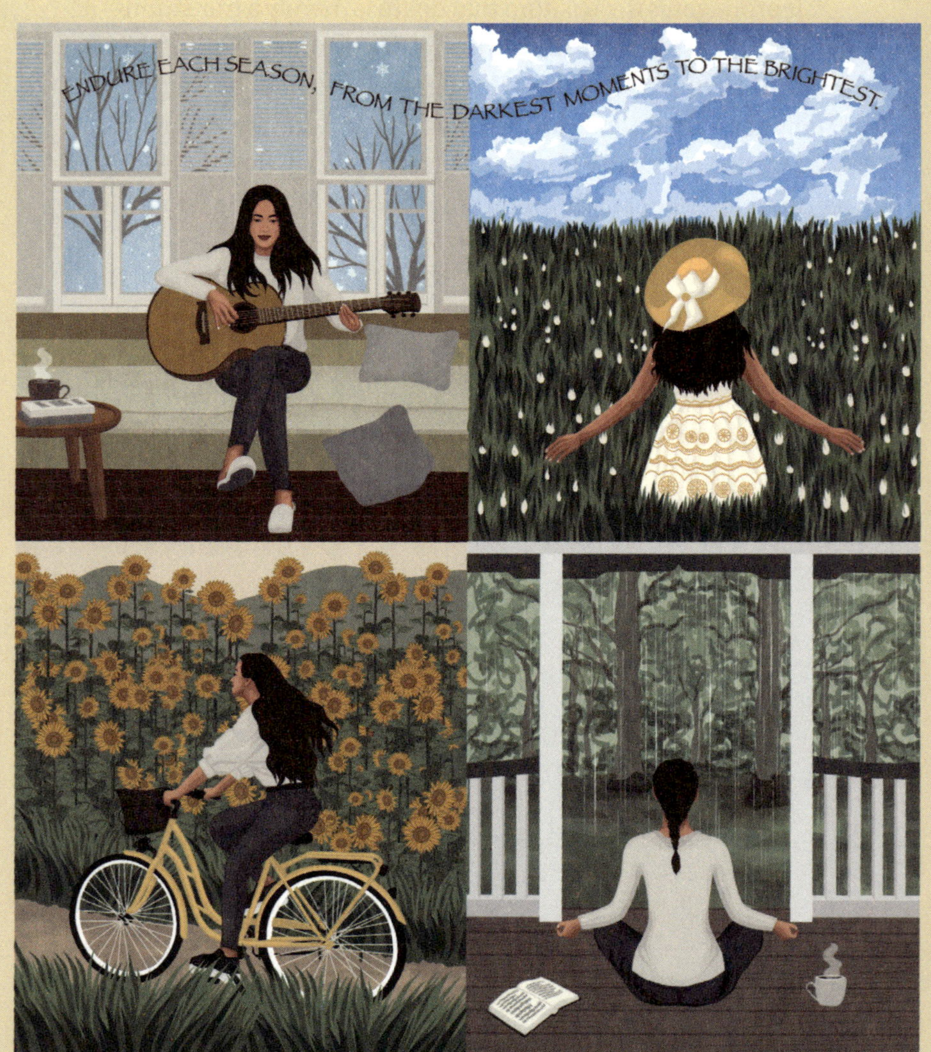
ENDURE EACH SEASON, FROM THE DARKEST MOMENTS TO THE BRIGHTEST.

2

INNER SEASONS

'Winter is statuesque in beauty,
Spring is vibrant,
Summer is energy to reckon with, and
Monsoon is a mosaic of them all!'

—ANONYMOUS

Have you ever wondered why there are certain days in a month when you feel super productive and over the moon, while on some other days, you feel gloomy and weary? Have you ever pondered the correlation between your emotions and the phases of the month? Have you ever thought how your emotions can resonate with different seasons? If such inquiries arouse your intrigue, then you possess the ideal disposition to comprehend the extraordinary synchronization between humans and the nature.

Merely examining the cyclical changes in weather, one can discern a deliberate pattern that not only sustains ecological harmony but also introduces diversity, fostering adaptability within the biosphere. The varying seasons serve as nature's mechanism to prevent stagnation, encouraging growth, renewal and a perpetual sense of change. By observing this interplay, it becomes evident that seasons are an essential component, breaking the monotony of life and contributing to the resilience and vitality of the natural world. Nothing can evoke profound emotions in humans as Mother Nature does. The four seasons—winter, spring, summer and monsoon—correspond with each other and influence vegetation, climate, flora and fauna necessary for human existence.

These four seasons are broadly linked to the four phases of the menstrual cycle and by simply modifying your habits to sync with each season, you can live in harmony with your hormones.[19] Besides, the change in seasons can also influence symptoms of menstruation, metabolism and mental health. Together, these variables determine the comprehensive growth of a woman, prompting a shift in our perspective towards our monthly cycles.

WOMEN AS NATURE

Prakriti (or nature) is often referred to as 'Mother Earth' because of its life-giving and nurturing qualities.[20] Nature is always fair and impartial; it procreates, blooms, feeds, protects and transforms to enrich the soil for plants. Similarly, a woman symbolises Prakriti, as she too governs the process of creating, nurturing and encouraging a life in her womb. We, as women, need to acknowledge and embody the concept of mirroring Mother Nature by following her design as nurturers.

In the modern age, women often face difficulties in balancing their work, home life, relationships and responsibilities. This can potentially result in burnout and may subsequently lead to health issues, including reproductive and emotional imbalance. To mitigate these challenges, it's crucial for women to develop a deeper connection with nature and understand the intricacies

[19]Fitzgibbons, Lucy, 'Phases of the Menstrual Cycle: The 4 Seasons,' *Lucy Fitzgibbons Naturopath*, 2 November 2020, https://www.lucyfitzgibbons.com/articles/phases-of-the-menstrual-cycle-the-4-seasons.

[20]'Prakriti,' *Britannica*, https://www.britannica.com/topic/prakriti.

of their menstrual cycles in order to maintain good physical and emotional well-being. In reclaiming their passions, they must navigate a path beyond mere duty, finding liberation from self-imposed restrictions.

INNER CYCLES

Many women suffer from painful menstruation; hence, understanding the reason behind the distress becomes a key requisite for the betterment of reproductive health. An underlying health issue can be understood by gaining insight into one's physical disposition, as nature has provided the tools required to treat them effectively.

This chapter will shift your perception of menstrual health and guide you in aligning with Prakriti for menstrual wellness. Every woman's experience of her inner seasons varies greatly, despite the cycles being inevitably connected to nature's spirited rhythm in innumerable ways.[21] Comprehending the workings of the four phases of the monthly menstrual cycle—menstrual, follicular, ovulatory and luteal—can help in gleaning the best out of each season with much ease and grace.

Phase 1: Menstrual Phase/Inner Winter (Days 1–5)

'In the midst of winter, I found there was,
within me, an invincible summer.'

—ALBERT CAMUS

[21]'The Inner Seasons of the Menstrual Cycle', *Red School*, https://www.redschool.net/blog/the-inner-seasons-of-the-menstrual-cycle.

Looking Inward

Winter, as we all know, is the coldest season of the year, and a mystical phase where we tend to restrict physical activity, embracing slower and more inactive lifestyles.

Furthermore, the bleeding phase entails a woman slowing down and finding refuge in herself, making this inward period one of the most insightful times of the month for self-reflection and healing. Symbolically, nature ensures that the Earth is planted with seeds until it is time for them to sprout and thrive when the rejuvenating spring finally arrives.

Biologically, menstruation is the phase women go through to complete nature's unfinished task of not being able to fertilize an egg in the womb. It is the phase when oestrogen and progesterone hormone levels drop, often leaving women feeling melancholic. These low-spirited emotions are called menstrual blues or the winter blues and are responsible for feelings of gloom, sadness and listlessness.

These symptoms can affect the mind negatively and impact the functioning of the reproductive hormones, especially if one is weary or experiencing other health issues. Failing to address these discomforts by identifying the root cause through introspection, nourishment and the right balance between rest and work can inadvertently disrupt the natural flow of periods.

By prioritizing self-care, women need to consciously recuperate from the feelings of being unproductive during this low-energy phase. Be mindful, as this phase is temporary. It is perfectly acceptable to rest but it is not advisable to sleep or lie down on the couch the whole day. Let this phase guide you to develop a positive attitude towards menstruation and support the healing process.

The inner winter cycle is the time when nature bestows upon you, as a woman, the freedom to recoup in the warmth of your inner sanctuary, despite external pressures to remain productive. Women need to seize this moment to care for themselves and listen to their hearts, allowing their visions—dreams, aspirations and the essence of their true selves—to surface and re-evaluate their priorities. Use this time to gain insights into your personal journey, fostering a deeper connection with your innermost aspirations and refining the path ahead.

While this winter phase not only assists you in shedding menstrual blood, it also helps discard the old and undeserving patterns by planting seeds for new beginnings and new goals.

Honouring your body's shifting needs will help you enjoy optimal health and wellness throughout your cycle. Every season serves its purpose; winter is the time to reschedule strenuous workloads and commitments, especially for habitual workaholics and energetic extroverts. Women must set boundaries and prioritize self-care during this inward, intuitive winter time.[22]

Trust Mother Nature to take you through brighter and more productive seasons ahead, giving you a new lease of life. Your winter mantra should be 'Rest, Recoup, Rejuvenate'.

Phase 2: Follicular Phase/Inner Spring (Days 6–11)

'The beautiful spring came;
and when Nature resumes her loveliness,
the human soul is apt to revive also.'

—HARRIET ANN JACOBS

[22]Geertsen, Lauren, 'How to Use Your Period for Intuitive Superpowers', *Empowered Sustenance*, 4 October 2018, https://empoweredsustenance.com/period-intuition.

Looking Outward

Inner spring or the pre-ovulatory phase occurs during the second week of the menstrual cycle, starting from day 1 of periods until day 14 and ends with the ovulatory phase. Spring succeeds winter and precedes summer; therefore, it becomes a time of new beginnings, when fresh buds bloom, hibernating animals awaken, birds build nests, new seedlings sprout and the Earth comes alive again. Similarly, this pre-ovulatory period gives rise to feelings of optimism and enthusiasm, bringing in a fresh, new outlook towards life.

With spring comes a gradual rise in oestrogen levels and FSH hormones, filling you with outward energy. Even the uterus gets busy planning and rebuilding its endometrial wall in anticipation of a probable pregnancy. Naturally, the woman's body is permeated with activity, making this an ideal time for productive endeavours. Support this follicular season by nurturing your body with balanced and nourishing foods.

Spring adds new enthusiasm to life. With hormones gaining momentum, it brings fresh perspectives and new interests to all aspects of life—be it career, relationships, educational pursuits or new challenges. After the winter slumber, the awakened mind feels highly motivated and inspires you to be a part of all ongoing activities.

The influx of hormones naturally makes one feel rushed. Hence, you need to plan consciously and diligently. Alleviate winter woes by rejoicing in the pleasantness of spring. Try not to let go of this 'plan and progress' phase by procrastinating. Enjoy the inner spring with all its wonder, without rushing things, as you are going to be pulled into the vivacity of the next phase.

Your spring mantra should be 'New Plans, New Learnings and New Endeavours'.

Phase 3: Ovulatory Phase/Inner Summer (Days 12-19)

''Cause a little bit of summer's
what the whole year's all about.'

—JOHN MAYER

Communication, Collaboration and Collective Action

Inner summer, or the ovulatory phase, occurs during the third week of the menstrual cycle and is considered the most fertile time of the month. Summer is a season of bright sunshine, abundance and prosperity, when the sun encourages and attracts everyone to step out and make the most of their time. This season offers you boundless physical stamina and should be harnessed by manoeuvring yourself in a productive manner, with peaking oestrogen levels encouraging outward action.

The brain's chemistry during this phase evokes feelings of generosity and inclusiveness, making it the best time to leave your comfort zone and shed inhibitions. The inner summer establishes a period of peak productivity for handling team projects, brainstorming new ideas, developing new interests, learning new skills, excelling at your job and nurturing relationships.

But women need to be aware that this phase may also make them experience heightened sexual drive as the body is preparing itself for a probable pregnancy. The escalating hormones will make you feel sensual. The body temperature rises and the cervix softens, which are nature's ways of encouraging procreation.

However, inner summer represents much more than just a physical expression of love and the sharing of intimate sexual energy between two individuals. This feeling goes beyond the surface, instilling trust, respect, confidence and self-esteem, creating a deep connection that allows emotionally connected partners to glimpse into each other's souls.

Sadly, in today's society, the focus has shifted from establishing meaningful bonds and profound aspects of intimacy to fixating on physical attraction and momentary pleasure.

The essence of warmth, grace and unity in intimate relationships is replaced by power dynamics and financial pursuits, often seeking fleeting satisfaction. This transition has, at times, resulted in emotionally taxing and detrimental connections with oneself and others.

The hectic pace of modern life leaves little room to form deep intimate connections—a tragedy in a technologically connected world that desperately needs human-to-human contact.

So be conscious of people with whom you share sexual power or intimacy, as an exchange of powerful energies during sex can either drain or elevate your feminine energy. Hence, it should be treated as sacred and not merely as a physical act.

In *The Arts of Seduction,*[23] narrative practitioner Seema Anand, who is an acknowledged expert on the *Kama Sutra,* advocates using the ideas of the *Kama Sutra* to engage the mind, share humour and enjoy cultural experiences. She believes that sex is sacred and has the potential to elevate the human mind, consequently leading to greater compassion and harmony in the world. Thus, individuals should consciously connect through sacred sex for a higher purpose in life.

Anand's book promotes a healthy attitude and wisdom towards sex and seduction, eloquently intersecting the

---

[23] Anand, Seema, *The Arts of Seduction,* Aleph Book Company, New Delhi, 20 June 2018.

historical and contemporary elements of everyday life. I believe this is more applicable to adults who are in a committed relationship.

Hence, during this phase, women must prioritize building their lives creatively and constructively and abstain from unduly indulging in material pleasures, as focusing solely on unhealthy obsessions, such as food, sex and material pleasures, may lead to exhaustion and depletion of energies, which can manifest as PMS in the following phase. Failing to balance work, rest, hobbies and self-care can confuse the body and trigger unwarranted emotions.

Hence, one should stay grounded, with clear perceptions, and take care of the gut by consciously including cruciferous vegetables, healthy proteins, antioxidants and fibre-rich foods that can make this season immensely productive and pleasant.

Your summer mantra should be 'Speak, Socialize and Shine with Cognizance'.

Phase 4: Luteal Phase/Inner Monsoon/Fall (Days 20–26)

'Life isn't about waiting for the storm to pass...
It's about learning how to dance in the rain.'

—VIVIAN GREENE

Unwinding and Grounding

The inner monsoon or the luteal phase refers to the final phase of the menstrual cycle when our bodies are preparing for the onset of a new bleeding phase. This is the phase when the progesterone hormone peaks but then plummets to its lowest point along with oestrogen in the absence of pregnancy. This sudden decline in hormone levels results in both the body and mind requiring time and space to recuperate.

The monsoon rain, much like the inner monsoon in a woman, brings life-sustaining elements to the surface. The rain replenishes the Earth with fresh potable water, crucial for the survival of all living beings. However, just like the heavy rains can cause soil erosion, a woman's inner monsoon can bring forth tumultuous emotions and hormonal fluctuations, leading to sadness, irritability and anxiety. The monsoon rain may be relentless, but with the right approach, a woman's inner monsoon can be navigated to foster recovery and renewal.

We need to be cognizant of these subdued emotions, which can otherwise disrupt our state of mind, routines and relationships by sending out wrong signals. If not addressed promptly, these emotions can contribute to a complex condition known as pre-menstrual syndrome that can result in physical and psychological symptoms due to extreme shifts in reproductive hormones. Ayurveda recognizes PMS as menstrual irregularities that can be addressed by holistic treatment methods.[24]

Seasonal change can be challenging for everyone. Psychologists say that fall is the season that gives an opportunity to consciously let go of negative thoughts of senseless ego, greed and pride, even if opportunities may look enticing, bright and colourful—just like fallen leaves. Readjusting commitments and workloads with patience and perseverance is the most impactful step we can take to avoid hormonal upheaval.

When our hormones are low and unsupportive, nature provides solutions through constant reminders that these complicated symptoms can be managed by maintaining a structured lifestyle to preserve our energy. A wise and assertive

[24]'Manage PMS with Ayurveda,' *School of Ayurveda and Panchakarma*, 24 June 2022, https://www.ayurvedacollege.net/blogs/manage-pms-with-ayurveda.

woman will develop the courage to speak up for herself and create healthy boundaries without getting pressured by the actions of people and situations.

Self-care is the way forward to enhance the body's natural rhythm. Furthermore, we should incorporate healthy practices by engaging all five senses to ground ourselves, such as yoga, breathwork, nature walks and boosting immunity with magnesium-rich foods.

Additionally, indulging in aromatherapy massages, having soulful conversations with supportive individuals and emphasizing more on activities that will act as stress-busters are all proven to be excellent ways to tackle PMS symptoms.

Maintain a journal and be watchful of indulging in sugar-laden foods, consuming alcohol and caffeine as well as staying up late. Unhealthy lifestyle habits have the power to unsettle the natural rhythm of your hormonal functions.

This season is an opportune moment for self-reflection by offering gratitude and showing appreciation for all that has been achieved; most importantly, by reassessing unfulfilled aspirations with acceptance and humility.

Make this season purposeful by extending kindness and offering a helping hand to those in need. This period of introspection can bring about a newfound understanding of the past, present and future, leading to fresh perspectives and opportunities. Consequently, the reward will be a less painful or pain-free menstrual cycle that uplifts your spirits and rejuvenates you. The phenomenon of the falling leaves serves as a symbol of the inevitable change, urging us to mature and grow with time, akin to the autumn leaves.

Your monsoon mantra should be 'Ground Yourself to Explore Your Inner World.'

'We cannot stop the winter or the summer from coming.
We cannot stop the spring or the fall
or make them other than what they are.
They are gifts from the universe that we cannot refuse.
But we can choose what we will contribute to life
when each arrives.'

—GARY ZUKHAV

THE BOTTOM LINE

Menstrual cycles are a part of the wheel of time. The fluidity of seasons is an ace example that the highs and lows of life are temporary and that hope is the only constant factor we need to hold on to throughout our lives. The extremities of cold, rain, fall, heat and wind take the lead during different seasons, and discomfort occurs only when we try to attach ourselves to one particular season.

Winter comes seeking patience, and spring emerges with a plan, giving way to the action-oriented summer and eventually conceding to the downpour of rain or the fall.

Embracing each season with all its wonder, flaws and blessings while learning to gracefully move from one phase to the next marks the beginning of a new and meaningful life.

NIMMI'S MANTRA

Embrace the natural rhythms of the seasons and stay attuned to your body to elevate your feminine energy.

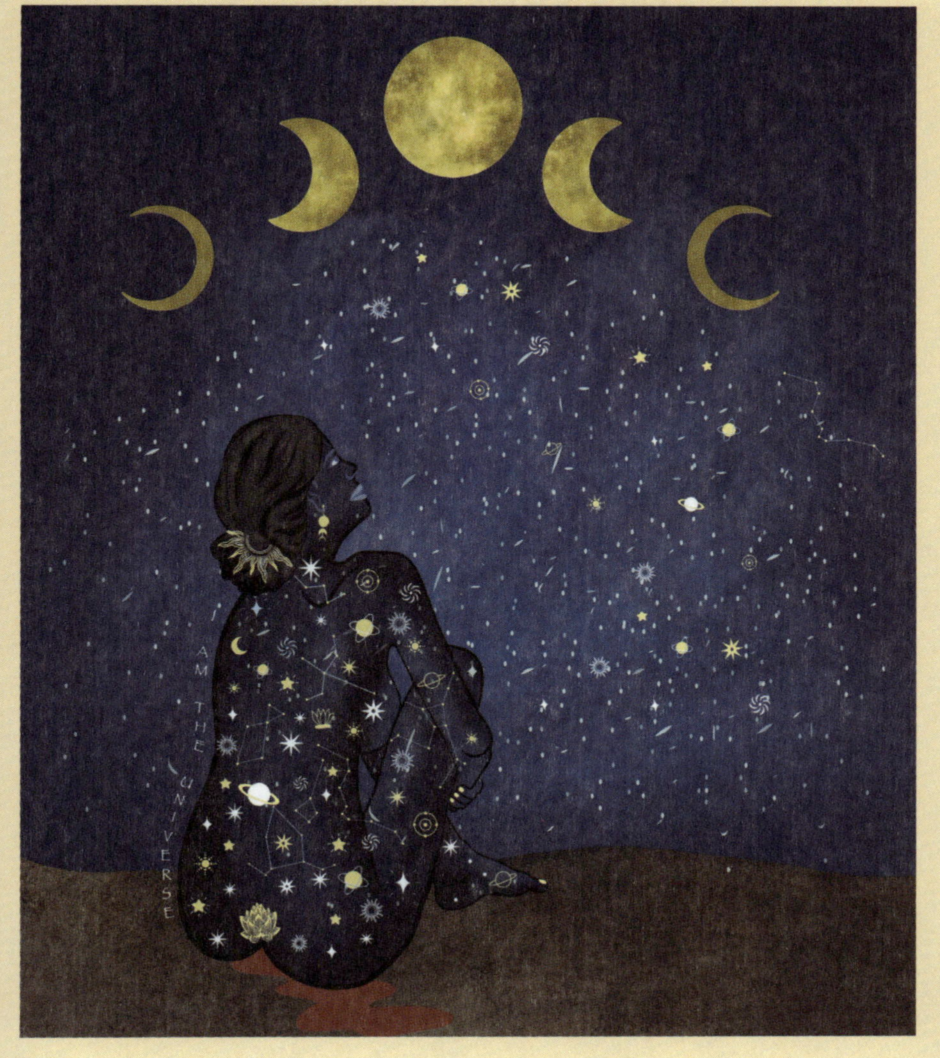
I AM THE UNIVERSE

3

THE LUNAR CYCLE

'And just like the Moon, you shall go through phases of light, of dark, and everything in between. And though you may not always appear with the same brightness, you are always, always whole.'

—MOLLIE BYLETT

Have you ever gazed at the full Moon on a clear night and pondered why our ancestors revered it as a symbol of femininity? Have you ever stood in awe of its ethereal and enigmatic aura in the night sky? Or did you ever consider that the phases of the Moon are believed to unveil the many facets of women, otherwise enshrouded in the lunar rays?

MOON MYTHOLOGY

Since time immemorial, humans have been observing the immaculate orbit of our cosmic partner around the Earth and its powerful effect on its inhabitants. Reports around the world reveal that the Moon's influence may also have been a major factor in making life on Earth possible.[25]

The study of human behaviour impacted by the lunar

[25] Lotzof, Kerry, 'How Does the Moon Affect Life on Earth?,' *Natural History Museum*, The Trustees of The Natural History Museum, London, https://www.nhm.ac.uk/discover/how-does-the-moon-affect-life-on-earth.html.

cycle dates back thousands of years.[26] Early humans believed that the Moon has a considerable hold on the human psyche, fertility, menstruation, birth rate, etc.; a few of which have been confirmed by modern-day research. People from primaeval Greece and Rome revered the Moon and gifted women crescent-shaped amulets and totems as they believed that these charms protected them from the evil eye. Devotees of the Moon from various cultures and traditions draw a spiritual connection between the Moon and menstrual phases.

The Moon has also been mentioned in ancient Hindu texts of *Ayurveda, Kama Sutra, Khagola Shastra* (Indian Astronomy) and *Jyotihshastra* (Hindu Astrology), which reveals that India has a strong and deep-rooted association with the Moon.

According to Hindu mythology, Lord Chandra, the Hindu God of the Moon, was cursed by his 26 wives (the other Nakshatras) to lose all his shine and gradually fade away, as punishment for favouring his love towards one of his wives Rohini.[27] The story follows that Lord Shiva helped Lord Chandra regain his brilliance by granting him the boon of coming back to life through the process of waxing and waning every month for the benefit of mankind. This is also the reason why a crescent moon adorns Lord Shiva's mane.

Even today, many Hindus follow the lunar calendar, where the months begin and end on a New Moon Day. Hindus believe that the lunar cycle is symbolic of the principles of life—birth, growth, maturation and death. Such references from early folklore to modern medicine reveal the strong influence of the Moon on humans.

---

[26]'Can the Moon Affect our Health?', *Royal Museums Greenwich*, https://www.rmg.co.uk/stories/topics/can-moon-affect-our-health-behaviour.

[27]Dalal, Roshen, *The Religions of India: A Concise Guide to Nine Major Faiths*, Penguin Books India, New Delhi, 21 April 2014.

GRAVITATIONAL POWER

The Moon is located approximately 3.8 lakh km away from the Earth. It is our planet's only natural satellite and is responsible for stabilizing the Earth on its axis with the help of its gravitational power. One orbit around the Earth brings about four different phases of the moon—the new moon (dark moon), the waxing half moon (first quarter), the full moon and the waning half moon (last quarter); these phases are visible to the naked eye.

The journey of the Moon, ascending from the new moon to the full moon is known as the waxing phase, whereas its descent from the full moon back to the new moon is called the waning phase. This journey around the Earth happens once every 29.5 days and is called the lunar cycle, which indicates that the Moon has completed one orbit around the Earth.

For ages, humans have observed the Moon exerting a strong gravitational pull on the Earth's oceans and the seas, and the ocean's tides rising in tune with the Moon's proximity to the Earth. The Moon and the Earth's water bodies interact with the electromagnetic fields of human bodies and subsequently affect us psychologically and physiologically.[28]

MENSTRUAL SYNCHRONY

'The moon taught me there is beauty
in darkness too, that even when
I don't feel whole, I am enough.'

—MARINE ASHNALIKYAN

Our universe holds countless secrets that are beyond human perception. Before the era of doctors, scientists and technologies,

[28] Clark, Dean, 'Are We Moonstruck?,' *Time and Date*, https://www.timeanddate.com/astronomy/moon/moon-effect.html.

the lunar cycle was considered a representation of the woman's periodic cycle and was often referred to as the moon cycle. The term 'menstruation' by itself means 'month of the moon', and is derived from the Greek word *mene*, meaning moon, and the Latin word *mensis*, meaning month.

Many people observed that the average menstrual cycle, with its 28–29 days period, and the monthly moon cycle, with its 29.5 days waxing and waning cycle, are almost in synchrony. This amazing similarity is the universe's way of demonstrating how women are blessed with the ability to live according to the rhythm of the sacred cycle of their wombs.

Throughout history women's menstruation has always been considered highly potent. Traditionally, women have treated menstruation as the awakening period of their inner Goddess', and permitted themselves to rest and recoup during this time. Resting, in ancient times, was not considered a stagnation to the progress of life but rather withdrawing from the outside world consciously. This process of aligning the celestial orb with their inner moon inspired many women to discover their true potential and emerge as better versions of themselves.

Long before the rise of patriarchy, there seemed to have been a profound and seemingly unbreakable bond between women and the Moon. They were known to collectively bleed with the new moon and ovulate with the full moon.[29] In some matriarchal societies, women who lived amongst nature in smaller tribes menstruated and ovulated around the same time and in sync with the lunar cycle. Those curious to delve deeper into this philosophy can refer to the McClintock effect (also known as menstrual synchrony).[30] It explores the concept

[29]Cohut, Maria, 'Menstrual Cycles and Lunar Cycles: Is there a Link?', *Medical News Today*, 12 February 2021, https://www.medicalnewstoday.com/articles/menstrual-cycles-and-lunar-cycles-is-there-a-link.

[30]Watson, Kathryn, 'Period Syncing: Real Phenomenon or Popular Myth?',

that women living in close proximity gradually experience more synchronized menstrual cycles.

Women are reawakening their femininity by venerating the Moon through modern rituals, becoming conscious of the workings of their womb. One such example is the resurgence of the ancient 'Red Tent' tradition.[31,32] This is a time-honoured ritual practised during menstruation when bleeding women would retreat to 'Moon Lodges' to rest, rejuvenate and exchange wisdom.

Traditionally, these women would retreat from their partners and children and gather in designated Red Tents, collectively talking about cycles and bleeding, sharing their personal experiences, embracing their intuitive abilities, reflecting on being a woman and bonding under the Moon's influence. The entire community honoured this tradition of women stepping away from their responsibilities to revive their inner feminine power.

Meanwhile, men eagerly awaited their return to receive insights arising from the intuitive powers of bleeding women. These messages encompassed aspects of health, work, relationships, marriage and children, which were received with humility for the well-being, progress, wisdom and prosperity of the entire community. Such has been the mysterious synchrony between women's menstrual phenomenon, men and the Moon.

Although the scientific community remains indecisive about the potential synchrony between the Moon and the

---

Healthline, Healthline Media, 23 January 2019, https://www.healthline.com/health/womens-health/period-syncing.

[31]Olorenshaw, Vanessa, 'The Red Tent Movement and a Circle of Women', *HuffPost*, BuzzFeed, Inc, 4 September 2016, https://www.huffingtonpost.co.uk/vanessa-olorenshaw/the-red-tent-movement_b_8091348.html.

[32]'Introducing the Red Tent Movement', Moody Month, https://moodymonth.com/articles/introducing-the-rent-tent-movement.

natural process of menstruation,[33] the Moon does hold an undeniable connection with one's moods, sleep, eating patterns and even love life, as stated earlier, guiding humanity with its mysterious presence. When the Moon has such a strong influence on humans, how can it not influence a woman's menstrual health? Sadly, modern society does not prioritize meaningful rituals, nutrient-rich foods and a much-needed balance between rest and responsibilities. People confine themselves to closed environments, work for prolonged hours under artificial lights and are constantly exposed to excessive stimuli from gadget usage. These harmful transgressions in lifestyle have led to heightened emotions, fears, anxieties and competition, particularly among the youth, far surpassing the experiences of older generations. Hence, modern women need sustainable healing tools and rituals to improve their menstrual and mental health.

MOON JOURNALING

Moon journaling is a powerful tool that provides an opportunity to work with celestial events in order to thrive and grow consistently.[34] Journaling your deepest feelings at various phases of the Earth's nearest celestial neighbour will aid you in maintaining mindfulness regarding your choices, supporting hormonal variations throughout the month with a clear perspective.

Regular journaling can help manage versatile issues such as menstrual or infertility problems, relationship issues, grief,

[33]Ziomkiewicz, Anna, 'Menstrual Synchrony: Fact or Artifact?,' *Human Nature*, Vol. 17, No. 4, 2006, 419–432. https://doi.org/10.1007/s12110-006-1004-0.

[34]Charters, Claire, 'Moon Journalling: Timing Your Intentions with the Lunar Cycle,' *Botanical Trader*, 4 November 2021, https://botanicaltrader.com/blogs/news/moon-journalling-timing-your-intentions-with-the-lunar-cycle.

addictions, coping with traumas and illness, etc. Synchronize your menstrual cycle with the moon cycle and awaken your divine feminine energy in the following way:

- Start gazing at the Moon as a ritual to become more aware of its distinct phases.
- Download a moon journal app on your phone or buy a moon journal with a printed calendar and write down your feelings.
- Create a private space for journaling.
- Have an internal dialogue, and if you have any worries or problems, write them down alongside probable solutions. Just putting your thoughts on paper can help you declutter your mind and align the pattern of your feelings with the lunar cycle. For example, jot down the behavioural patterns of your moods during a particular moon phase and your menstrual cycle and note down everything (people or situations) that drains or lifts your spirits.
- Reflective writing helps in expressing difficult emotions and being aware of your feelings. This can help identify negative feelings like fear, anger, anxiety or sadness that may be caused by hormonal variations or due to unpleasant situations or people.

Journaling as a self-care ritual can change your perspectives and motivate you to take action and overcome the biggest hurdle in your path, which is 'You.' However, every woman's menstrual cycle and fertility are negatively impacted due to artificial light, working long hours and leading a sedentary lifestyle. Regular journaling over a period of time can instinctively establish patterns that will direct you towards your exclusive book of dos and don'ts.

PHASES OF THE INNER MOON

'If women used to cycle with the moon
Did we all used to be in sync
Keeping the world's rhythm inside ourselves'

—NIKKI TAJIRI

Women go through four distinct hormonal phases just like the Moon every month. The Moon's phases are classified into the new moon, waxing moon, full moon and waning moon, while a woman's monthly cycle is divided into the menstrual, follicular, ovulatory and luteal phases. The four lunar phases and four menstrual phases are fluid and open to interpretation. The more women embrace their inner moon, the more advanced and comprehensible the womb's mystical connection with the celestial body, and this meaningful connection encourages women to harness their unique femininity, embracing it as a source of strength and empowerment. Let us now uncover the mysteries of this celestial orb and decode the messages it holds for the millions of women experiencing different phases of menstruation.

Phase 1: Inner Moon Phase/Menstrual Phase—Healing and Recouping

'In the stillness of the dark moon, we find
the power of silence and the wisdom of surrender.'

—ANONYMOUS

The 'dark moon' or new moon is considered as the first week of the menstrual cycle and is symbolized as the 'emergent life force.' The nature of the dark moon is to seek a new lease of life. Allow this dark phase to assist you in releasing old and undeserving patterns alongside the shedding of menstrual blood and letting go of anything that no longer serves you.

The Universe is cautioning you to be attentive and seize the moment, to set positive intentions for every desire prior to starting a new project, relationship, health plan or hobby. Now is the time to envisage solutions to heal fertility and menstrual issues by visualizing that they have already transpired. It is also wise to keep all intentions and future plans under wraps until they begin to take shape.

Your uterus works hard to shed its menstrual blood. So you may feel drained of energy and spirit. You must develop a habit of not being available to the outside world by indulging in self-care; be more attuned to your inner feelings. The new moon phase is a period of healing and self-reflection, with the cynosure being rest and consuming nourishing food. Make sure to be a passive observer as this habit can equip you to be super productive and adventurous in the phases to come.

Just as the Moon grows bigger and brighter with time, your seed of intentions also grows and manifests into a full-grown tree in due course.

In this fast-paced modern world, it's important to set intentions mindfully and to proceed with patience, awareness and vigilance as they guide you towards a life filled with wisdom, clarity, solutions and abundance.

Moon Guidance from the Universe

- Turn inwards to develop an intuitive mind.
- Set intentions for your goals and aspirations to manifest them into reality.
- Be compassionate to yourself by honouring the inner dark moon.

Phase 2: Inner Waxing Half Moon Phase/Follicular Phase—Trust and Hope

'Oh, Maiden Moon, now hear my plea,
hearken, hearken unto me!
As you grow, my spells enhance,
and power its magic with your dance.'

—ANONYMOUS

The waxing half moon is the dynamic phase that represents the second week of the menstrual cycle. After darkness, there always comes light. This is Nature's way of conveying that the darkness of the Moon or the bleeding phase will end and give way to the brighter moon. During the follicular phase, as hormones responsible for building the uterine lining increase, the Moon also gradually grows larger, symbolizing the natural progression of fertility and renewal.

This phase is characterized by outward energy, and women's plans and aspirations experience exponential growth. Those who are forthright often attract opportunities, exuding social enthusiasm for new ideas. These sentiments mirror the waxing moon's eager progression towards the full moon stage.

Be prepared to give shape to all goals and thought processes that were, until the previous week, deeply buried as a seed in your subconscious. The stronger your motivations towards your goal during the dark moon phase, the more they blossom during the waxing phase. Be fearless and take the leap of faith into the unknown. Be liberal in setting intentions that attract joy, love, wealth, health, universal guidance and wisdom.

Make sure to remain alert and mindful of any opportunities that come knocking, as this is the time to widen your network and move forward with confidence. However, be vigilant and wary as the rising energy levels can make one over-optimistic and result in burnout. It would be wise to cultivate patience and perseverance while moving forward to experience the full force of the coming phase—the bright full moon.

Moon Guidance from the Universe

- Believe in yourself.
- Plan and progress.
- Be disciplined and stay committed to moving forward.

Phase 3: Inner Full Moon Phase/Ovulatory Phase—Actions and Celebration

> *'And just like the Moon, we must go through phases of emptiness to feel full again.'*
>
> —ANONYMOUS

Of all the phases, the full moon is the brightest and the most insightful period for women. This is the third phase of the menstrual cycle and is packed with powerful energy. The inner moon sparks a flurry of activity within a woman's body and mind, making this ovulatory period emotionally vibrant and sensual. However, it can also leave you feeling emotionally vulnerable. This is the phase where women reap the rewards for the intentions set during the dark moon period, as they manifest into reality.

With the peaking hormones, your outward masculine energy is also soaring high, making you feel powerful, dynamic, inclusive and sensual. Your spirited feminine energy makes you generous, nurturing and compassionate. Thus, seize the moment, expand your horizons and express yourself. Take advantage of opportunities to socialize, plan important meetings, start new projects, address unresolved issues and more.

Studies show that this is also the most fertile time of the month for those inclined towards motherhood.[35] With the Moon fully bright and shining, women are emotionally wired with a brighter and more positive frame of mind, accommodating and celebrating life.

You must conclude all high-energy activities with clarity, displaying the maturity and wisdom that come with this phase. This is the ideal time to bridge your inner emotions with outer world experiences and reinforce self-trust. Detach yourself from unpleasant thoughts and past experiences by listening to your intuition. Further, conserve and sustain your energy by gradually reining in ego-driven, achievement-oriented masculine energy that helps you finish tasks. Focus on nurturing feminine energy at the end of the phase to avoid burnout, as nature has its own rules and hormones have their limitations.

This deliberate shift helps you to embrace the softer aspects of your being, fostering creativity, intuition and inner peace. By doing so, you prepare yourself for the cycle to begin anew, equipped with a deeper understanding and respect for your body's natural rhythms and the wisdom it imparts.

Moon Guidance from the Universe

- Foster collaboration over competition by building meaningful connections with others.
- Engage in self-care practices to revitalize your senses and rejuvenate yourself.
- Graciously acknowledge the attainment of previously set goals and aspirations.

[35]Soumpasis, Ilias, Bola Grace, and Sarah Johnson, 'Real-life Insights on Menstrual Cycles and Ovulation Using Big Data,' *Human Reproduction Open*, Vol. 2020 No. 2, 2020, hoaa011, https://doi.org/10.1093/hropen/hoaa011.

Phase 4: Inner Waning Half Moon Phase/Luteal Phase—Reflect and Release

'And the moon said to me—my darling daughter,
you do not have to be whole in order to shine.'

—NICHOLE MCELHANEY

As the full moon descends from its high pedestal and transitions towards the waning phase, the inner moon diminishes its energy, moving towards darkness and emptiness. The last phase of the menstrual cycle invites you to turn inwards; observe and re-evaluate all your intentions, ideas, investments and relationships, which may or may not have worked out in the previous intense and fast-paced phases.

Be watchful, as hormones can excite the mind and bring out certain character traits that are typical of PMS. This waning phase can release high-strung energy and may prove to be destructive. So take note of this transition period, which holds hidden messages to the darker side of the woman's psyche, bringing valuable lessons to the forefront. This is the ideal time to cleanse and detoxify the body while working on unresolved emotional blocks. Pay attention to physical symptoms, such as migraines, anxiety, sleep disturbances, low libido and sugar cravings, to identify the right emotions behind them. This metamorphosis is the first step towards strengthening your health.

Over-exertion or excitement can lead to frustration, irritability and anger, which are the most common emotional indicators of PMS, and leave you with a sense of discontentment. This is the phase to reflect on developing an inner sense of peace and a heightened state of focus. Recognize that you cannot be an energetic superhuman at all times, nor can you constantly shine bright like a full moon. During this phase, it is preferable to finish ongoing tasks rather than starting new assignments.

You should also make an effort to shed old patterns. Move forward from toxic situations or relationships while being grateful for the lessons learned, as they can help you uncover a new version of yourself. Spend time in solitude to reflect and declutter both thoughts and spaces. Prioritize self-care, which can avert repercussions spilling into the next cycle.

Let this creative waning phase help you with its boons of heightened intuition and creative abilities to stay grounded. Set aside some time for yourself by stepping away from your family or loved ones to foster a deeper connection with your inner self.

Extend help to those in need with a grateful heart. As the Moon wanes, becoming smaller and darker, you too go through phases of emptiness to feel full again.

Moon Guidance from the Universe

- Embrace the power of letting go, and allow yourself to release pent-up emotions and stress.
- Redirect your focus towards productive endeavours that bring you joy and fulfilment.
- Take time to reflect on the darker aspects of your life and find gratitude for what you have and the experiences that have shaped you.

Being open to the subtle messages from each phase and harnessing them receptively can bring in favourable results and amazing transformations physically, mentally and spiritually.

THE RED AND WHITE MOON CYCLE

Our ancestors delved deep into understanding a woman's power and the mystical connection between menstruation and the Moon. They revered women who menstruated with the new moon as 'White Moon women' and those with the full moon as 'Red Moon women.'[36,37] Ancient traditions worldwide honoured both White Moon women and Red Moon women for their distinct qualities. Society acknowledged and embraced their vital roles in looking after both the spiritual and material welfare of the people.

The White Moon Cycle

'The strongest women become the strongest mothers before their children are even conceived.'

—ANONYMOUS

Women menstruating around the new moon and ovulating during the full moon were traditionally associated with the White Moon cycle. Our ancestors regarded the full moon phase as the most fertile period on Earth. Women aligned with the White Moon cycle were believed to have optimal chances of conception. As such, they were revered as fertile, nurturing and compassionate, and were considered guardians of progeny.

The traditional White Moon women were portrayed as nurturing, caring, protective and emotionally driven towards family life. They exuded maternal energy, dedicating themselves to the upbringing of their children. White Moon women were often the guardians of tradition and culture. Despite the changing times and highly competitive world of today, the White Moon women still embody these nurturing qualities, whether they choose to be homemakers, entrepreneurs, artists,

---

[36]The white moon cycle refers to when menstruation occurs during the new moon and ovulation occurs during the full moon, whereas the red moon cycle indicates bleeding during the brighter moon phase and ovulation during the new moon.

[37]Craft, Christie, 'What is Sacred Menstruation? Here's How to Reclaim Your Period,' *Nylon Entertainment*, 26 November 2015, https://www.nylon.com/entertainment/red-moon-cycle-full-moon-period.

astronauts or CEOs. The essence of her power remains in her innate nurturing tendencies and her ability to bring comfort and care to those around her, fostering a sense of warmth and security in their lives.

The Red Moon Cycle

'She is the enchantress of beauty
That every soul would love to adore.'

—ANONYMOUS

Women who menstruate on the full moon and ovulate on the new moon were known to be in the Red Moon cycle. Historically, these women were the natural healers of the tribe and were called 'medicine women,' witches, enchantresses, priestesses, conservationists and bearers of magic and wisdom.[38] They were considered to have a deep desire for self-actualization and focused on channelling their creative energy inward.

Our ancestors recognized the tremendous power of women who could create and sustain life. These wise women used their innate powers to heal, preserve and guide the community. They recognized the power of menstruation and encouraged other women to channel their energies towards a greater cause, while also standing up against unjust authoritarian culture.

However, in medieval times, these powerful women were often labelled as witches and persecuted for their feminine power. Today, the Red Cycle women play a vital role in the world as global leaders, entrepreneurs and mentors. They have the potential to lead with grace and dignity and are considered to be mature maternal figures who guide and shape the future

[38]Jay, Shani, 'Sacred Bleeding: White Moon & Red Moon Cycles Explained,' *Revoloon*, https://revoloon.com/shanijay/052020-white-moon-and-red-moon-cycles.

of the community. Despite facing challenges, these women remain passionate and outgoing and dare to maintain their vulnerability. Their mission is to make a positive impact on society and be a beacon of hope for others.

In addition to archetypes of women belonging to the white and red moon cycles, there exists a fascinating realm known as the 'wise woman cycle', where women seamlessly transition between both cycles, each imbued with its distinct purpose. Such women impart their unique, valuable and powerful energies by playing their roles effectively based on their temperaments and purpose of existence. It is fascinating that these women can experience the gifts and wisdom of both cycles. Regardless of the cycle you find yourself in, give your body what it needs and do what feels good for the soul.

THE MOON BATH RITUAL

Engaging in rituals to elevate energies can bring peace and stability to a wandering mind. During the full moon or the new moon, the lunar energy is at its peak, and participating in simple practices can help to block negativity and align one's vibrational frequency with their true nature and soul in the following manner:

1. Set up a sacred space and bring in the fire element to cleanse it by lighting natural or organic aromatic candles or incense.
2. Create a zen-like setting by playing soothing music to calm high-strung nerves.
3. Gadgets have a way of muddling one's senses and are best kept away during such healing and renewing processes.
4. Add half a cup of pink salt; a quarter cup of Epsom salt, magnesium sulphate or bath salts; six drops of essential

lavender or jasmine oil; and a few rose petals or jasmine flowers into a tub of warm water. Soak yourself in it for at least 20 minutes.

5. Epsom salt baths enhance relaxation and decrease muscle fatigue or soreness. Relax and reflect by taking a few deep breaths.
6. Silently chant positive affirmations. Be grateful for all that is being served to you during the full moon and the new moon phases. Acknowledge any negative emotions or feelings that need to be addressed.

Alternatively, you can record your aspirations on a piece of paper, place it under a sealed bottle of water and allow it to soak up the Moon's energy overnight. In the morning, drink the charged water with gratitude and reverence as this can amplify your intuitive abilities. Our bodies are comprised of 60% water, on average, and the Moon represents the water element, so drinking this charged water aligns you with its transformative energy and empowers you to manifest your deepest desires.

To manifest powerful intentions, it takes 21 days of consistent effort and alignment with the Universe. This can be achieved by syncing with the lunar energy and making positive changes in your thoughts and behaviour. Here are some ways to tap into the power of the Moon:

1. Reframe your thoughts and speak positively about menstruation.
2. Keep track of the lunar cycle and adjust your schedule accordingly.
3. Engage in moon journaling to reflect on your personal growth.
4. Meditate while gazing at the moon to cultivate inner peace.

5. Observe fasting during the new moon and full moon phases.
6. Balance your rest, leisure, nutrition and work with the changing Moon phases.
7. Embrace the transformations brought by each phase.
8. Let go of any habits, beliefs or memories that no longer serve you.

THE BOTTOM LINE

Aligning the Moon and menstrual phases can strengthen and sharpen your intuitive mind to confidently navigate through unchartered waters. It unceasingly communicates, with those who can decode the silent messages, via journaling, moon meditation or rituals. Resonating with the different phases of the Moon can bring about immense improvements to the self, which can be observed in personal growth, menstrual and mental health, education, career, relationships and coping skills.

NIMMI'S MANTRA

Just as the Moon goes through phases of waxing and waning, we too must experience periods of emptiness to fully appreciate and find fulfilment in life.

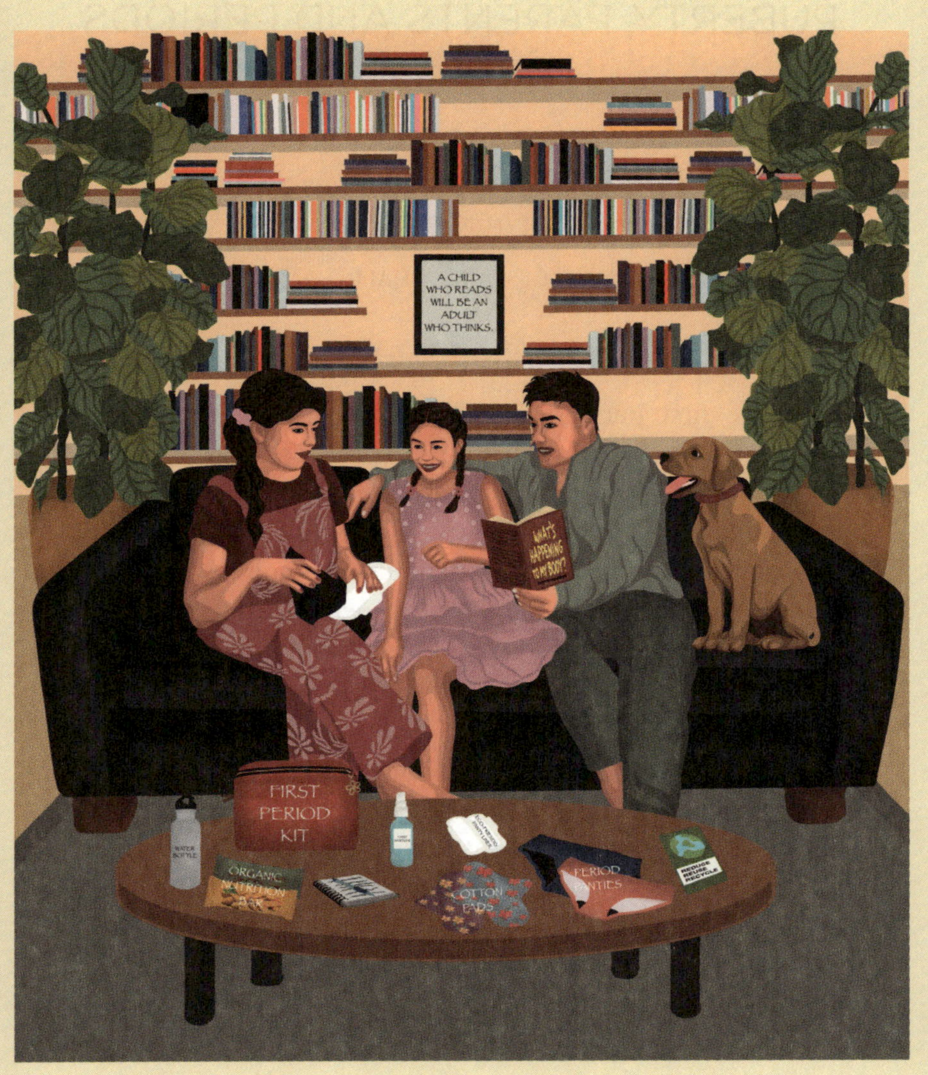
A CHILD WHO READS WILL BE AN ADULT WHO THINKS.
WHAT'S HAPPENING TO MY BODY?
FIRST PERIOD KIT
WATER BOTTLE
ORGANIC NUTRITION BAR
COTTON PADS
PERIOD PANTIES
REDUCE REUSE RECYCLE

4

PUBERTY, PARENTS AND PERIODS

'Puberty for a girl is like floating down a broadening river into an open sea.'

—G. STANLEY HALL

The first period, also known as menarche, marks a significant milestone in the life of an adolescent girl. It is a mystifying phase, symbolizing her blossoming into womanhood as she begins her first menstrual cycle. Puberty is a stage marked by myriad of confusing emotions, awkward moments and conflicting thoughts, which understandably cause parents to be anxious and protective of their children. Each child encounters certain challenges in their journey to reach adulthood.

This chapter serves as a valuable resource for parents concerned about the changes taking place in their daughter's life. It provides insights into the reasons behind these transformations and offers solutions to facilitate a meaningful and memorable transition from childhood to adulthood.

PHYSICAL AND CHEMICAL CHANGES

During puberty, the pituitary gland releases LH and FSH into the bloodstream. These hormones are found in both males and females, though the way in which puberty manifests differs greatly between the sexes. In females, LH and FSH prompt the ovaries to produce reproductive hormones, including oestrogen and progesterone, preparing the female body for adulthood. These hormones are accountable for the thickening of the uterine lining.

Hormonal Turnaround

The mantra echoing within a girl's body during puberty is 'hormones, hormones and more hormones'. A whole set of new chemicals are activated within her body, facilitating her transition into her teenage self. This release of hormones manifests physically and emotionally, making the adolescent phase of her life exciting but equally taxing.

The hormones that are responsible for the 'good, bad and ugly' interventions take place during this phase. These hormones play a significant role in shaping various physical and emotional changes. Some of these changes include a sudden growth in height and weight, the appearance of pubic and axillary hair, the development of breast buds, vaginal discharge and acne breakouts.

Puberty also brings about internal emotional developments, such as mood swings, sudden changes in energy levels, increased fatigue, heightened attraction and curiosity about the opposite sex, an obsession with appearance, sugar cravings and behavioural transformations, which may cause a shift from being an extrovert to an introvert or vice versa. These changes vary in intensity between individuals, depending on the levels of FSH and LH hormones, which work relentlessly to enable the menstrual flow.

Preparing for Menarche

With expeditious changes in lifestyles, some girls might experience menstruation early—even as young as eight. There are numerous factors that can accelerate the onset of puberty in young girls, including hormone-laden food and dairy products, endocrine-disrupting chemical-infused cosmetics, decreased physical activity, excessive external stimulation and stress from 'digital overdose'.[39] Additionally, the lack of parental supervision in managing screen time adds another dimension to these concerns.

Contemporary research has reshaped our understanding of how fat tissue triggers a complex feedback loop that can accelerate the maturation process. This revelation, as articulated by Robert H. Lustig, M.D., a distinguished clinical paediatrics professor at the Benioff Children's Hospital, University of California, San Francisco, in his book *Fat Chance*, underscores a compelling connection.[40] It revealed that girls with a high body-fat exhibit elevated levels of the hormone leptin. This hormonal surge can act as a catalyst for premature puberty, consequently leading to increased oestrogen production. High oestrogen levels, in turn, foster greater insulin resistance, setting in motion a cyclical pattern wherein girls accumulate more adipose tissue, thereby boosting their leptin and oestrogen levels. This self-reinforcing cycle persists until they reach adulthood.

Puberty demands an incredibly compassionate approach from parents, as this transition can be daunting for a child. Despite many parents being well aware of the workings of adolescence, they might still feel helpless and overwhelmed when navigating their children's puberty.

---

[39] Bozzola, Elena, Giulia Spina, Rino Agostiniani, Sarah Barni, Rocco Russo, Elena Scarpato, Antonio Di Mauro, Antonella Vita Di Stefano, Cinthia Caruso, Giovanni Corsello, and Annamaria Staiano, 'The Use of Social Media in Children and Adolescents: Scoping Review on the Potential Risks', *International Journal of Environmental Research and Public Health*, Vol. 19, No. 16, 2022, 9960. https://doi.org/10.3390/ijerph19169960.

[40] Lustig, Robert H., *Fat Chance: Beating the Odds Against Sugar, Processed Food, Obesity, and Disease*, Avery Publishing, New York, NY, 31 December 2013.

'Each day of our lives we make deposits in the memory banks of our children.'

—CHARLES R. SWINDOLL

Based on my research and counselling experiences, I have outlined a few basic guidelines that parents can follow to ease the girl-to-woman transition.

1. *Start Young*

The understanding of the menstrual cycle cannot be attained as a crash course for a young girl. It must be imparted gradually, as the child matures both in mind and body.

Effective communication is key to promoting a healthy and natural understanding of the menstrual cycle in young girls. Start by having open and inclusive conversations about bodily changes from a young age, as early as six or seven years old. Engage with your daughter in playful talks about the workings of the womb and how every woman goes through this process. Use creative examples, such as birds, bees and pets, to explain the concepts of menstruation, hormones and bleeding in a simple and non-intimidating manner, ensuring she has a strong grasp of the natural process before experiencing her first period.

Guide her through dialogues that are practical and fact-based, before menarche, as she needs to feel secure about the changes and hormonal variations occurring within her body. Parents should engage in conversations with an open and pleasant frame of mind in order to provide the right understanding of the subject. Hence, discussions should be conducted during simple, everyday activities or while enjoying hobbies together. Gifting her an age-appropriate book featuring insightful illustrations can be enlightening, helping her comprehend her body and anticipate the changes she will undergo during this period. All these efforts from parents can empower a child's young and impressionable mind to challenge the cycle of menstrual stigma prevalent in society, ensuring she never has to whisper about needing a pad or a tampon or feel awkward to convey that she is on her period.

2. *Compassionate Parenting*

Due to hormonal fluctuations, adolescents experience new behavioural symptoms that may cause mood swings, sadness, desire to isolate, unhealthy eating habits, defiant behaviour or more extreme symptoms such as self-injury, suicidal thoughts and detrimental use of social media. An open and inclusive family setting can help adolescents navigate these emotions and parents must take care not to criticize their children or blame themselves for these hormone-induced thoughts. Instead, a safe space needs to be created for constructive conversations where young girls can voice their concerns about periods, menstrual product choices, natural pain relief options, understanding of sex, pregnancy, the opposite sex and mental health issues without any bias or prejudice.

Parents should start teaching their children the right names for sexual body parts using anatomically correct terms, such as vagina, breasts, uterus and ovaries, and encourage them to use these words appropriately.

Try not to be resentful about your personal experiences with periods around your young daughter so that they don't perceive menstruation as an as an embarrassing secret.

Young minds are impulsive, and hence following the mantra, 'Respond, Do Not React' can bail parents out from triggering any resentment. Remember never to react to their hormone-induced retorts with counteracting statements. Instead, calmly respond to them with clarity. Children have an inherent trait of learning and absorbing the actions of their parents and subconsciously registering them in their mental rule book. Be assured that there is no 'perfect parent' but a supportive one who appreciates and acknowledges the feelings that children share.

Puberty is also a phase of being exposed to situations that may cause embarrassment, such as unexpected first periods or blood staining one's clothes in public places. Hence, preparing a child in advance about such situations and offering practical solutions can instil confidence to handle natural and inevitable processes without feeling ashamed. While a child is struggling with puberty, a parent needs to proactively handle insecurities and temper tantrums with patience and perseverance.

Parenting is a lifelong commitment. Both parents need to redefine their relationship with their daughter with trust and respect in order to create a safe, stable and caring environment to explore her new identity. When these issues are addressed with commitment, they will positively shape your daughter's life, enabling her to thrive in every aspect of her life.

3. *The Dad-Daughter Duo*

'Behind every great daughter is a truly amazing dad!'

—ANONYMOUS

While both parents set the ball rolling for the physical, mental and moral development of their children, fathers play a significant role in their daughters' lives and set the foundation for shaping their personalities. A father holds a special place in his daughter's heart by being her first role model and trusted confidante. He plays a pivotal role in bolstering her self-worth and confidence, and perhaps most significantly, in nurturing a positive body image that stems from deep self-love.

A father's influence, especially during her formative years, becomes the template on which she sets her pattern for the future. As she grows older, the dad she hero-worshipped becomes a friend, philosopher and guide who helps to find her position in the world.

Thoughtful fathers speak respectfully about women without referring to their appearance or body type. They are aware that their daughters look up to them and observe how they treat their family members. A father who berates women for their body shape verbally or through non-verbal signs will result in the daughter developing a negative body image in her mind.

A father's emotional neglect or physical absence can develop feelings of abandonment in a daughter's life. It could lead to symptoms such as eating disorders, body shaming, self-doubt, getting attracted to emotionally unavailable partners, distrusting the masculine—all these traumas significantly affect emotionally, wounding feminine energy in her adult years.

A perceptive father who is physically and emotionally present at every stage of his daughter's development makes a world of difference, boosting her confidence and self-esteem. Girls having a stable family display more resilience in dealing with stress by maintaining balanced relationships and enjoying healthy interactions with both men and women. These young women develop life skills and attitudes, which lead to forming healthy relationships with men and choosing compatible life partners.

A girl's menarche marks a significant rite of passage, signifying her body's healthy alignment with the natural laws of the universe. A father's loving support and understanding can be instrumental in dispelling any potential shame or discomfort that may arise in the mind of a young woman during this time. In a predominantly patriarchal society, it is crucial for fathers to approach discussions about hormones and menstruation with openness and impartiality, creating a sense of normalcy by demystifying the menstrual experience.

A growing body of research highlights the powerful impact fathers can have on their daughters' mental well-being and emotional stability,[41] with their presence or absence having the ability to shape her psychological outlook throughout her lifetime.

4. *Body Positivity*

'In a society that profits from your self-doubt,
liking yourself is a rebellious act.'

—CAROLINE CALDWELL

Pooja Kochar, blogger and body-positive activist based in Mumbai, mentioned in an article that girls don't decide to hate their bodies, we teach them to.[42] How true this is! Many studies have shown that a negative body image is influenced by a multitude of external factors—the attitude of parents, peers, culture, institutions, digital and print media and childhood experiences.[43]

Adolescents face a wave of pressure and criticism from society but the pressure of having a perfect body and flawless skin surpasses all other expectations. The advertisements for beauty aids and make-up and slimming products create a false sense of reality through unrealistic and morphed images of women with a toned body and spotless skin, as portrayed

[41]Zia, Asbah, and Saima Masoom Ali, 'Positive Father and Daughter Relationship and Its Impact on Daughter's Interpersonal Problems,' *Journal of Social Sciences and Humanities*, 2018, 61–68.

[42]Kochar, Pooja, 'How These Girls Taught Me That They "Don't Decide to Hate Their Bodies, We Teach Them To",' *Youth Ki Awaaz*, YKA Media Pvt. Ltd., 29 January 2016, https://www.youthkiawaaz.com/2016/01/positive-body-image-in-young-girls/.

[43]Tort-Nasarre, Glòria, Mercè Pollina Pocallet, and Eva Artigues-Barberà, 'The Meaning and Factors That Influence the Concept of Body Image: Systematic Review and Meta-Ethnography from the Perspectives of Adolescents,' *International Journal of Environmental Research and Public Health*, Vol. 18, No. 3, 2021, 1140. http://dx.doi.org/10.3390/ijerph18031140.

in digital media. When those unreal results are not achieved after using the products, it severely impacts the self-worth of young, teenage minds. Young girls must be taught to accept their bodies and not follow a trend of unhealthy dieting or starving to have a 'perfect body' to fit into a dream dress.

Body shaming is gaining predominance in today's world, and it has become the norm to criticise aspects of others' physical appearance without a thought. Adolescents, being at their most vulnerable stage, become easy targets, falling prey to society constantly comparing them with others. This leads them to spend valuable time researching how to make their waists look slimmer and hide their imaginary flaws, further leading to shame, emotional fallout and, in some cases, suicidal thoughts.

Inculcating body positivity in younger minds begins at home. Parents must encourage their children to rightly interpret information and images presented in the media by filtering negative or misleading material. They need to have open discussions about unrealistic standards, superficial lifestyles and the pressure of social media. They should also clear their children's misconceptions about comparing themselves with celebrities and models, so that the latter focus on building their personality.

It is parents' responsibility to set the right atmosphere—by being their children's first example. Body positivity will improve children's mental and physical well-being, allowing them to focus on the quality of life with the best resources available.

Helping young minds focus on appreciating non-physical qualities, such as kindness, trustworthiness, caring, dependability and encouragement, can replace negative emotions with positive ones. Educating your daughter on body constitutions (*vata, pitta* and *kapha*), and inherent physical countenance can give her an insight into her unique genetic make-up, helping her to respect her body and that of others.

5. *Importance of Hygiene*

Menarche is the time when bodily secretions, such as sweat, oily scalp, acne, vaginal discharges and hormone-induced body odour, start manifesting physically. These secretions are a normal part of adolescent growth. However, ignoring proper hygienic practices can give rise to fungal infections, severe itching in private parts, urinary infections and foul-smelling discharges. If left unattended, these can harm our reproductive organs. Parents should realize that children may sometimes avoid expressing or addressing their concerns due to the fear of being shunned or teased by their friends and peers. These issues must be handled with care or they could lead to embarrassment and social withdrawal.

It is parents' responsibility to be alert and introduce their children to a daily routine of good personal hygiene. This can boost children's emotional quotient and make them feel more comfortable while interacting with people, easing their transition to adulthood with discipline, orderliness and self-esteem. Helping young girls understand their bodies and teaching them self-love will help them make sound decisions about their physical health and accept periods positively.

6. *Gift of Privacy*

Adolescence is a critical developmental period that requires both parents and the youth to redefine their relationships. This is the phase when children begin to explore themselves and traverse new avenues. They are catapulted into the field of sexuality and develop romantic relationships, as feelings of infatuation and love begin to form. Every day can be a battle trying to untangle their emotions of insecurity, anger, irritability and restlessness. All these are typical characteristics of adolescents and it is natural for them to desire some private space to work on their rapidly developing emotions and bodies. As they try to find their identities in this world, parents must ensure to give them space and privacy and trust for developments to happen at their own pace.

7. *White-collar Guidance*

Feeling vulnerable about their physical and emotional developments can force adolescents to withdraw into their shells.

Hormonal fluctuations coupled with a desire for approval can render some adolescents emotionally unstable. This vulnerability may lead them to succumb to addictive behaviours, including experimenting with substances like drugs, alcohol, etc., as the allure of exploration is particularly potent during this period.

There is also a plethora of problematic information available through unreliable sources that can greatly affect a young child's mind and their outlook on life. Here, parents need to step in to protect a child's well-being and virtues, avoiding criticisms and accusations that could leave scars for a lifetime.

To address parental concerns about their daughter's emotional well-being and their menstrual cycle variations, it is advisable to seek the assistance of school counsellors. Timely intervention and seeking guidance from professional medical practitioners, therapists or trusted relatives are crucial in directing young and fragile minds on the right path. This can significantly aid in their development of life skills.

Parents, in such pivotal moments in their daughter's life, hold the power to either impart wisdom and guide her through self-discovery, or let her grapple with an unsupportive societal narrative. At this juncture timely and open discussions with daughters become not only essential but also meaningful.

As a family, it is necessary to acknowledge the importance of mindful practices and rituals such as maintaining cleanliness in the house, reciting mantras or prayers, yoga sessions, sticking to regular meal times, helping in household chores and engaging in outdoor activities. Further, as a family, it is important to explore nature by embarking on safaris, visiting sustainable farms, venturing into the countryside, camping in tents, going on small treks and experiencing coastal camps. These activities not only offer a dopamine fix but also instil a deeper connection with nature, fostering personal growth and resilience.

In addition to outdoor activities, incorporating habits like reading intellectually stimulating material, practicing techniques for relaxation and breathing exercises can foster clarity and maintain peace within the family. These disciplined and simple routines can help build a child's emotional fortitude, enabling them to face life's challenges with strength and optimism.

Simon Sinek, esteemed author and motivational speaker, astutely observed that Millennials and Gen Z are often drawn to the dopamine-inducing rush of seeking social approval and engaging in online interactions.[44] In this relentless pursuit, they may inadvertently overlook the formation of meaningful relationships, potentially leading to mental disorders like depression and addictions later in life. This pattern can also result in a deficiency of crucial qualities such as discipline, patience, social skills and critical thinking.

Hence, it is of paramount importance to recognize that this isn't the youth's fault; they have come of age in the digital era where these dynamics are the norm. Therefore, it is the parents' responsibility to instil the right values and aid in developing strong character. Rather than imposing rigid rules upon them, they should serve as guides, encouraging them to explore a diverse array of experiences.

---

[44]Bilyeu, Tom, 'Simon Sinek on the Millennial Question,' *Success*, 10 January 2017, https://www.success.com/simon-sinek-on-the-millennial-question-2/.

A significant number of millennials and Gen Z are deeply impacted by technological advancements, especially the widespread use of the Internet and the proliferation of smartphones, which have had a profound impact on their lifestyles, communication habits and consumer behaviours. They hold a unique reverence for inclusivity, environmental consciousness and social justice, embodying an unwavering dedication to fostering equality and sustainability.

8. *The Holistic Way*

India is emerging as a global leader in traditional medicine and holistic practices such as ayurveda, yoga, herbalism, naturopathy and acupressure and medicinal oil massages. My humble message to every mother, mother-to-be and grandmother from different cultures around the globe is to make the most of holistic health practices by incorporating these into their routines with guidance from experts.

Consider celebrating menarche by involving all family members, if it aligns with your family's traditions and preferences. It is important to make way for meaningful rituals in which the old and young generations come together to honour, nurture and celebrate girls in a way that gives them confidence in life and makes them feel proud about their bodies.

9. *The 'Timeless' Period Bag*

Lastly, the most valued gift for every young girl about to experience puberty would be her first period kit. Parents cannot always be around but they can plan and prepare their daughter for any surprise. This period bag can become a security blanket for your daughter and save her from the embarrassment and trauma of getting a period in unexpected situations.

Here are a few pointers on the essentials that one needs

to think of while preparing a first period bag, which can be personalized as well:

- Two to three sustainable or eco-friendly pads for tweens
- Pantyliners
- Underwear or period panties and wet dry bags
- A hand sanitizer
- A pair of black tights
- Steel water container to combat headaches and cramps
- Healthy, organic nutrition bars (oats/millet, peanut/sesame), made of nuts and dry fruits or dark chocolate.
- A handy notepad to write down her thoughts on her experience of menarche.

Here are a few parental guidelines to ensure your daughter has a peaceful and joyful first period:

- Involve your daughter in choosing the right products for her period bag, and introduce her to healthier, sustainable and eco-friendly options, which can help reduce carbon footprints.
- Be prepared to assure her inquisitive mind with appropriate answers.
- Teach her how to use and dispose used pads responsibly.
- Talk about breasts, vagina, hair growth and periods in normal conversations, using the right biological words.
- Accept the fuss she might make during her periods. Allow her to complain without branding her behaviour.
- There are times when fluctuating hormones make it hard for a child to accept the rules laid down by parents. Labelling her as a 'rebel' can only complicate issues. Practise patience, restraint and tolerance during her emotional outbursts.
- Make a conscious effort to teach the importance of physical activities. Any form of exercise is ideal in today's digital age.

- Teach her the value of sharing with less privileged people in society.
- Keep reassuring your daughter of unconditional love throughout her turbulent teen years.
- Encourage her to set up achievable goals and help her in pursuing activities that she is passionate about.
- Hone her social skills and show her how to be responsible and accountable for her health.
- Allow her to see you as a kind, forgiving, responsible and helpful human.
- Encourage group or individual hobbies, such as yoga, music, sports, art, gardening, reading, debating, theatre and holistic rituals to keep her productive, flexible and grounded.
- Acknowledge her transition from childhood to womanhood through celebration.

By adopting and implementing these pointers, you will see your daughter develop into a successful woman.

THE BOTTOM LINE

L.R. Knost, award-winning author, feminist and social justice activist based in Florida, said, 'When little people are overwhelmed by big emotions, it's our job to share our calm, not join their chaos.' An adolescent can neither consider herself a child nor is she an adult. As she undergoes significant changes, parents are the most reliable people for their daughters to voice her frustrations. So bear with her, express concern, be supportive of her choices, stay calm and simply cuddle her to make this journey less conflicting. Remind her that every girl goes through this transition. Bring a smile and keep adjusting your little princess' crown along the way.

NIMMI'S MANTRA

Your girl's journey isn't about struggle, it's a transition. Help her through this transition and support her in experiencing a positive menarche.

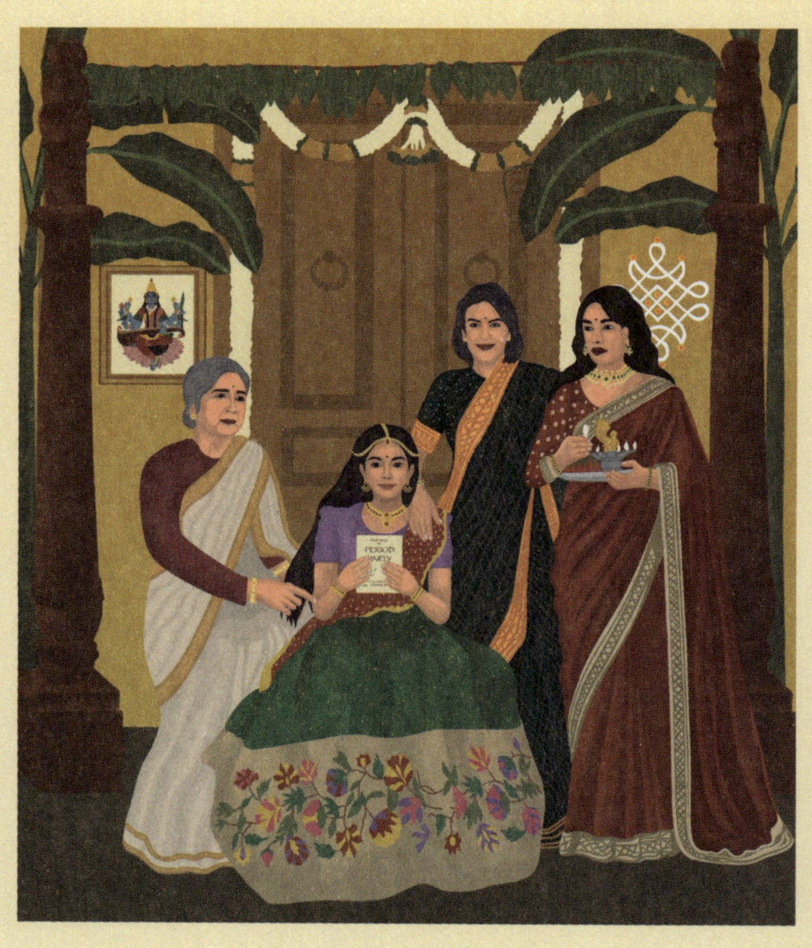
PERIOD
PARTY

5

MYTHS, MYTHOLOGY AND TABOOS

'At menarche, you meet your wisdom.
With monthly bleeding, you practice your wisdom.
At menopause, you become your wisdom.'

—TAMARA SLAYTON

For generations, menstruation has been shrouded in various myths and cultural beliefs. With the passage of time, this natural biological process has turned into a topic enveloped in taboo and silence.

In many cultures, menstruation is viewed as a private affair, whereas in others, it remains a widely discussed topic. Our early ancestors emphasized the significance of menstruation and honoured it in their unique ways. They were foresighted and discovered the secret to awakening the inner feminine goddess through the menstrual cycle. Therefore, the entire community celebrated menarche, the first occurrence of menstruation, with great veneration. Every country, culture and community governed by matriarchal tribes believed that nature and its five elements—water, earth, sky, fire and air—profoundly influence women's reproductive health and menstruation.

CELEBRATING MENARCHE

'Rituals are the way we mark the moments that matter.'

—DR CLARISSA PINKOLA ESTÉS

Menarche celebrations foster respect, encourage dignified conversations about periods, allow for an open dialogue and practice of meaningful rituals, nurturing a positive relationship with menstruation.

Research shows that tribes across the globe have historically celebrated and continue to celebrate this transition with ceremonies and rituals rooted in their indigenous culture.[45] From Australia to Europe and from Africa to Asia, menarche has been celebrated by every nationality, marking the significant transition of a girl into womanhood.

For instance, in Canada, the first period prompts a unique berry cleanse for young girls, who then spend a year gathering berries before consuming them to celebrate their passage into womanhood. Berries have antioxidants that help relieve menstrual cramps. In Ghana, a young girl is honoured with a regal celebration, where she is seated under a ceremonious umbrella and showered with gifts and blessings. In Japan, menarche is celebrated as a familial affair, with the mother delighting her relatives by presenting a traditional dish known as sekihan, which consists of sticky rice and azuki beans, symbolizing the announcement of the girl's maturity.

While it is interesting to know the diverse ways in which countries around the globe celebrate menarche, it is equally intriguing to explore how these rituals are honoured closer to

[45] Aquino, Leo, '5 Menstrual Rituals Around the World & What They Can Teach Us', *The Fornix*, The Flex Company, 23 October 2020, https://blog.flexfits.com/menstrual-rituals-around-the-world/.

home. India, with its vast expanse, is a rich tapestry of cultures and religions that have a multitude of customs and beliefs surrounding this significant rite of passage.

In comparison with other countries, India's menarche rituals have similar undercurrents, but with slight differences, emphasizing much-needed rest, nutrition and ceremonial feasts. The common thread across most South Indian states, however, is that grand celebrations mark a girl's first period.

In Karnataka, Tamil Nadu and Andhra Pradesh, the approach to marking this milestone is distinct, and is celebrated with a ritual known as the 'half-saree custom'. Also called the Ritu Kala Samskara ceremony or Ritushuddhi, the ritual involves donning a young girl in a half-saree as a way of announcing to the world that she has reached puberty, and half-sarees become the girl's attire at ceremonial events until her marriage when she puts on a full saree.

The half-saree tradition is not just a rite; it is a moment of pride and joy for parents. During the nine-day celebration, the menstruating girls are showered with nourishing delicacies like dry fruits, sweets made from pure cow ghee, and other treats designed to enhance their physical and reproductive health. To honour their menstrual cycle, the girls are given dedicated space for rest and relaxation, highlighting the importance of self-care.

The festivities culminate on the ninth day with a sesame oil massage, followed by a purifying bath using a mixture of neem and turmeric water. The girl is then dressed in traditional bridal attire, adorned with fine jewellery and a head full of jasmine flowers. The women of the family create a celebratory atmosphere, singing hymns, performing *aarti* and offering blessings and gifts. Similarly, in Kerala, menarche is celebrated as 'Thirandukalyanam' by the Nair community to honour and celebrate a girl's menarche.

These rituals are still adhered to in many rural and semi-urban South Indian households. However, the gradual decline in such celebrations is inevitable as the main intention of this custom earlier was often to signify that a girl was of marriageable age soon after menarche.

In North India, girls go through menarche without much fanfare or celebration as menstruating women are confined to their homes to rest.

In Assam, Tuloni biya is a tradition similar to a wedding, where a girl is married to a banana plant instead of a groom and smeared with turmeric paste, given a ceremonial bath and bestowed with gifts from family and friends.

It is admirable how these communities embrace celebrating a natural event, often viewed as forbidden, but true benevolence extends beyond this initial rite of passage. It lies in ensuring that a girl does not endure isolation during her periods for the rest of her life, fostering a lasting sense of respect and support.

The current trend of first period parties in urban areas endeavours to break down societal taboos. However, engaging in open discussions about menstruation is crucial to destigmatize this natural aspect of female physiology, fostering understanding and promoting a healthier perspective on menstruation.

Christiane Northrup, M.D., said, 'All indigenous people on Earth provide their young people with specific rites of passage to signify their change in status from child to young adult.'[46] The customs of menarche celebrated in many countries is a prime example of this.

In today's world, many households around the globe honour and celebrate their daughters' first period to build period-positive mindset.

---

[46]Northrup, Christiane, 'Celebrating a Girl's First Period,' *Christiane Northrup, M.D.*, 20 November 2006, https://www.drnorthrup.com/celebrating-a-girls-first-period/.

Preserving these rituals are crucial as these practices would set an example for their younger siblings and eventually their daughters and granddaughters.

EXPLORING MENSTRUAL TABOOS

'All females deserve menstrual well-being,
and that includes knowledge and reassurance
about her body from the earliest possible age.'

—NIKKI TAJIRI

In ancient times, prior to the domination of patriarchal beliefs and the widespread influence of Christianity, women were revered as sacred beings and menstruation was viewed as a transformative spiritual experience. Our foremothers recognized the divine potency of menstruation and deemed it necessary to cultivate this power through rituals of solitude and introspection for the benefit of the community.

Menstruation is a crucial aspect of reproductive health that deserves to be openly and positively discussed, both among women and men. It is vital to break down the barriers of taboo and ignorance.

Patriarchal systems worldwide have perpetuated the misconception that menstruating women are unproductive and hinder societal progress. They deemed discussions of normal menstrual topics inappropriate or uncomfortable and collectively excluded women from participating in all socio-economic aspects of life, as many men feared the power of femininity.

This systematic ostracization made women feel ashamed and apologetic for experiencing a natural, biological phenomenon, severely damaging their psyche and warping their attitudes towards menstruation for generations. Such gender-based discrimination is rightfully challenged by the modern and educated women of today. Women are focusing on building their careers for financial freedom, allowing them to break free from patriarchal constraints and associated traumas. Consequently, this has also influenced men's perspectives, who are now increasingly engaging in more open and healthy dialogues regarding menstruation.

We must recognize that our early matriarchal ancestors never considered menstruating women as 'untouchable,' but emphasized that they should rest and recuperate, requiring seclusion to awaken their feminine power. Many menstrual rituals, though thoughtfully established, evolved and faded due to misinterpretations or dilutions of truth by the uninformed over time.

Our ancient traditions and rituals have often been misconstrued and misinterpreted, but it is crucial to rectify them today in order to restore confidence and positive acceptance of menstruation among the present generations. Echoing the Western world blindly is another reason for many to treat these customs as a hushed affair. Regardless of East or West, as part of a progressive society, it's imperative not to create negative consequences for future generations.

Healthy menstruation is a vital component of progress, and it is the collective responsibility of society, regardless of cultural or geographical differences, to embrace it. The only way to counter contemporary ignorance and hatred towards menstruation is to educate ourselves and future generations with the right mindset. For instance, one can explain the concept of rituals as a process of primary care rather than imposing them as rules, which could be detrimental to a young girl's emotional health.

Modern society has made significant progress in accepting and honouring menstruation, as shown by the gaining popularity of Red Tents and Moon Lodges worldwide. They are proving to be beneficial not only for rest and recuperation but are also a special space for women to hone their skills related to self-care, holistic well-being, creative expression and rituals that contribute to personal and collective empowerment. These might involve activities like mindfulness, storytelling, herbal knowledge, artistic pursuits or any practices that enhance mental, emotional and spiritual well-being. The exact skills can vary widely depending on the individual and specific focus of the community or gathering. Embracing self-care without resisting their own bodies, particularly during menstruation, becomes a transformative journey towards healing. This path has the potential to yield purpose and productivity in subsequent phases.

Every ritual has a scientific reason behind its success. However, if the same ritual is practised without a suitable reason, it can create confusion and have a negative impact on younger generations. Hence, it is imperative that rituals are explained logically, with accompanying scientific facts.

MYTHS AND FACTS

'Your personal mythology is the loom
on which you weave the raw materials of
daily experience into a coherent story.'

—DAVID FEINSTEIN AND STANLEY KRIPPNER

Myths are unverified claims that are yet to be proven scientifically. However, they might contain elements of truth. I am sure everyone has grown up experiencing their share of myths around menstruation, which have existed for hundreds of years but often have some logical reasoning behind them.[47]

[47]Puneeth, Dr Sanmathi, 'Menstruation—Myths and Facts,' *Health Vision*, https://healthvision.in/menstruation-myths-and-facts/.

Some common myths include avoiding pickled food during periods, sleeping on grass mats, not entering the kitchen and avoiding visiting temples. Below are a few theories intended to enlighten everyone about the rationale for these practices:

Theory 1: Avoid pickled food

Consuming pickled food during the menstrual cycle can negatively affect gut health. The high levels of salt and spices in pickles can lead to bloating and cramping, which results in digestive discomfort. Avoiding pickled items during this time is advisable to maintain good health and minimize discomfort.

Theory 2: Sleep on grass mats

Mats made of *kusha* (*Desmostachya bipinnata*) grass, commonly known (in English) as Halfa grass, are considered sacred and have medicinal properties. Sleeping on kusha mats helps to control cramps and acts as a natural coolant. Research says that kusha grass is also used as a medicine to treat urinary disorders and dysmenorrhea.[48]

Theory 3: Avoid entering the kitchen

In traditional joint families, women were required to do a lot of manual work. During menstruation, elders advised them to abstain from their regular chores, including socializing, practicing rituals and worship, and rest as a means to recoup and rejuvenate.

Theory 4: Avoid visiting temples

Places of worship are built for reasons. In Hindu culture, it is believed that visiting a sacred sanctum helps elevate the body's

[48]'Kusha (*Desmostachya bipinnata*) Uses, Research, Medicine, Side Effects', *EasyAyurveda.com*, https://www.easyayurveda.com/2017/10/05/kusha-desmostachya-bipinnata/.

energy from a lower to a higher level for growth and abundance. However, for menstruating women, it is believed that energy is concentrated in lower levels and moves downward, facilitating the shedding of blood from the uterus. Thus, visiting the sanctum during menstruation may disrupt the body's bioenergy and hormonal flow. This theory can extend to chanting and other religious practices, potentially causing conflicting energies during menstruation.

Noted author Sinu Joseph, an educator who has dedicated her life to creating awareness about menstrual health, in her popular book *Rtu Vidya* has shattered misconceptions surrounding menstrual health.[49] Her dedicated research in rural India reveals the reverence of age-old customs among Hindu women, who embrace their role as guardians of the tradition and believe in the benefits of menstrual rituals for reproductive health.

She explains the various causes behind customs and traditions, which should be recognized as the wisdom of our forefathers. Their foresight has undoubtedly led to numerous advancements in the present day, underscoring the enduring relevance of these time-honoured practices in shaping our cultural tapestry and guiding future generations.

MENSTRUAL GODDESSES

Hindu culture has always revered goddesses and their supreme power. Deities like Lajja Gauri—featuring the Goddess lying down with her legs spread, representing the womb at the moment of birth—and Parvati—where her idol at the Chengannur Mahadeva Temple in Kerala undergoes menstrual bleeding—embody the sacred feminine in their entirety. Notably, the famous Kamakhya

[49] Joseph, Sinu, *Ṛtu Vidyā: Ancient Science Behind Menstrual Practices*, Notion Press, Chennai, 25 September 2020.

Temple in Assam, which dates back to the eighth century, is devoted to the menstruating Goddess Kamakhya Devi, who is revered as the bleeding goddess and is also synonymous with intense feminine power and fertility.

According to the ancient scripture, the *Kalika Purana*, after her nuptials to Lord Shiva, Goddess Sati first experienced her menstruation at this holy site. Another legend holds that during Shiva's devastating dance with the body of Sati, the womb or yoni of the goddess fell at this temple, transforming into the revered deity Kamakhya.

Kamakhya is a Shakta Tantric deity, who is regarded as the Goddess of Desire. In June every year, this temple offers a red cloth (symbolizing the Goddess' menstrual blood) to all its devotees, including men. It is mind-boggling that a centuries-old temple has a ritual through which the devotees receive symbolic 'menstrual blood' cloth as blessings. This tradition honours menstruation in the land of Gods and Goddesses. We are a society deeply rooted in a rich culture and we still appreciate ancient celebrations with the sole intention of celebrating women.

Menstruation Across Cultures: A Historical Perspective by Nithin Sridhar dispels misconceptions regarding menstruation.[50] This book serves as a revelatory guide, especially for individuals with an open mind and a drive to construct flourishing communities.

WOMB HEALTH DEFINES GENERAL HEALTH

Most women menstruate between their menarche and menopause, marking this as the most integral period of

[50]Sridhar, Nithin, *Menstruation Across Cultures: A Historical Perspective*, Vitasta Publishing Private Limited, New Delhi, 25 December 2018.

their lives. This journey includes several challenges such as puberty, pregnancy and motherhood, and involves major physical and emotional upheavals. Women deal with these challenges whilst facing discrimination from both men and other women. It must be stressed that all complications related to menstrual health greatly affect a woman's mental, physical and social well-being. Hence, women must consciously develop self-compassion, have a sound knowledge about menstrual irregularities and maintain a balance between various activities.

In Ayurveda, it is believed that during menstruation, there is an emphasis on supporting the downward flow of vata, or the 'wind' element, through practices such as rest, nourishment and quietude. These practices aim to promote balance and comfort during menstruation, acknowledging the body's natural processes and energy flow. Additionally, staying hydrated and engaging in gentle movements or yoga tailored to support the body during this time are also commonly recommended in Ayurvedic tradition.

THE BOTTOM LINE

History shapes our existence, making it the responsibility of every individual to broaden the vision by accessing the right kind of information based on research and facts and educating the younger generation. Thus, preparing a young girl for the sacred journey of menstruation, creating a safe environment and weaving a web of support is crucial. Women serving as positive role models play a pivotal role in helping young girls uncover their feminine wisdom through meaningful rituals.

NIMMI'S MANTRA

Broaden your vision towards menstruation, for it is in the celebration of your blood that life will reveal its profound significance to you.

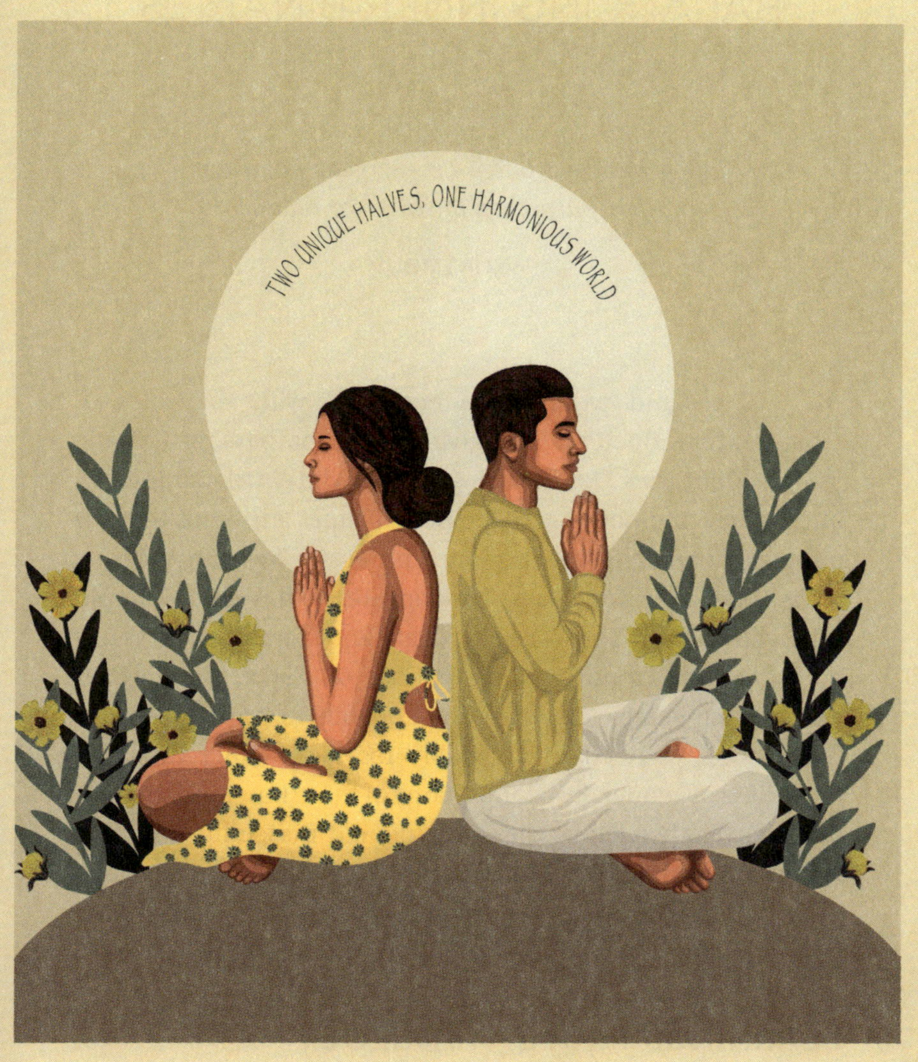
TWO UNIQUE HALVES, ONE HARMONIOUS WORLD

6

BALANCING INNER BINARIES

'Life is designed based on energetic polarities,
and our purpose is to strive for balance.'

—ANONYMOUS

Men and women are entrusted with the roles of reproduction, caregiving and harnessing cosmic energies. Despite being created with equal importance, intelligence and power, they possess distinct attributes that are unique to their genders. A common phrase we've heard growing up is 'Men are from Mars, Women are from Venus.' I would urge you to shed your Martian coats and remove your Venus tiaras, as you are not separate entities on Earth. The Earth is for all living beings to coexist and cohabit. To bring about this realization, we need to invariably reset our inner dualities, regardless of gender. By taking charge of these inner binaries, we can effortlessly balance the feminine and masculine energies, fostering harmony without unnecessary conflict.

I hope this chapter sparks your interest in understanding your dualities, paving the way for a more fulfilling life.

LEARNINGS FROM MYTHOLOGY

Ardhanarishvara, as depicted in Hindu scriptures, is a half-masculine (Shiva) and half-feminine (Shakti) form merged in the middle. Devi Shakti, or the sacred feminine, unites with Lord Shiva, one of the principal Hindu Gods, and is portrayed as Ardhanarishvara. This embodies the delicate balance between *Purusha* and *Prakriti,* the respective masculine and feminine energies of the Universe. These dualities (Shiva Shakti) hold the key to human life, and their seamless integration as Ardhanarishvara serves as a potent metaphor for the importance of balancing opposing energies, such as knowledge and ignorance, light and darkness, consciousness and unconsciousness, to maintain cosmic equilibrium.

Delving deep into the concept of Ardhanarishvara, ancient texts define prakriti as the body and mind, with all its constitutional parts, and purusha as pure and egoless consciousness that governs life and reality. Nature emphasizes that both prakriti and purusha embrace each other's true nature and flow rhythmically, like the days and seasons of the Earth.

The dualities present in nature are omnipotent. Nature teaches us how essential it is to balance the uniqueness of our own nature to find peace.

Purusha, or masculine energy, represents the physical realm and is action-oriented, whereas the feminine energy prakriti represents creation, imagination and intuition. Every woman's spiritual realm connects the man's logical mind with his heart. Together, they balance, regulate and manifest the Universe's creative process.

Prakriti takes immense satisfaction in creating and nurturing, as she is the body and mind while purusha is the free spirit who passively watches over prakriti. His real being steps in in times of chaos, confusion or a threat to his existence.

Similarly, the Taoist symbol of harmony, yin and yang, represent dualism—the belief that all forms of energy have an equally powerful, opposing energy.[51] Indeed, life is a balancing act and is most fulfilling when we learn to embrace dualities in all their forms—joys and sorrows, summer and winter, death and birth, movement and stillness—with grace and gratitude.

Here is a fundamental insight from our ancient scriptures depicting both the masculine and feminine energies evolving and merging as one, embodying the true essence of nature.

FEMININE ENERGY

'A woman in harmony with her spirit
is like a river flowing.
She goes where she will without pretence
and arrives at her destination
prepared to be herself
and only herself.'

—MAYA ANGELOU

Women by nature are the feminine/yin energy—emotional, compassionate, nurturing, vulnerable, receptive, flexible, creative, artistic and explorers of the darker side of life. Compared with a river, she keeps flowing, sometimes sweeping gently and sometimes rapidly, reflecting the inherent qualities of femininity. Like the river, women possess a dynamic and nurturing force that shapes the landscape of life.

Prakriti is the potent force that creates a beautiful environment for future generations to thrive in. The evolving nature of womanhood (prakriti) is undergoing a metamorphosis in the present day, as women are rising as formidable, dynamic

[51] Kostin, Anastassia, 'Balancing Act: How Yin Yang Promotes Harmony and Balance', *Pepperdine Graphic Media*, 1 December 2019, https://pepperdine-graphic.com/balancing-act-how-yin-yang-promotes-harmony-and-balance/.

and confident individuals. Education is igniting awareness and fostering new realms of freedom and responsibility. Women are transcending traditional roles, not only as homemakers but also scaling uncharted heights and asserting themselves in an array of decision-making roles. This progress is commendable. However, it is crucial for women to balance their masculinity with their inherent feminine energy to maintain menstrual and emotional wellness. The essence of a balanced life is to not find permanence in any single energy.

Supporting gender equality doesn't mean diminishing anyone; it is about uplifting everyone. It signifies that for a woman, other women are her allies while maintaining a harmonious relationship with men.

'Yes, I am a feminist, and feminism is for everyone' should be the prakriti mantra.

MASCULINE ENERGY

'The mark of a real man is a man who can allow himself to fall deeply in love with a woman.'

—C. JOYBELL C.

Men embody Yang (masculine energy)—characterized as rational, action-based, hunters, aggressive, protectors and providers. Society expects men to be steadfast, loyal and logical, holding them to high standards of wealth, power and success.

True masculinity lies in being compassionate and protecting and supporting the opposite gender. From a young age, men should be taught to be empathetic towards women. It is crucial for a man to balance his inner dualities by constantly reminding himself that genuine manhood requires respecting women from all walks of life, being empathetic during their menstrual lows and celebrating their triumphs. A man displaying controlling, domineering or insecure behaviour reveals an imbalance in his feminine energy.

'Yes. I am a man of quality. No. I do not feel threatened by a woman of equal stature' should be the purusha mantra.

BALANCING INNER BINARIES

'A man does what he can;
a woman does what a man cannot.'

—ISABEL ALLENDE

Are you competing or completing?

It is essential for us to balance the masculine and feminine duality within us, for a well-balanced and structured society. While our inner masculine energy strives to race towards accomplishments, survival, freedom and power, our feminine energy wants to show love, be nurturing, be creative and express ourselves freely. If both these forces do not align, living our best lives remains an elusive goal. Hence, identifying our inner dichotomies and healing our inner child will bring clarity to our behaviours and help in moderating and balancing negative traits with ease.

At the core of a deeply fulfilling relationship lies the art of nurturing individuality, where each partner embarks on a journey of personal growth, leading rich and fulfilling lives of their own. This nurturing approach forms the bedrock of respect, trust and care, dissipating tensions and infusing the relationship with a vibrant and exhilarating energy.

Here is a simple way to distinguish between the positive and negative aspects of masculine and feminine energy to identify our inner dichotomies.

Negative or Wounded Masculine	Positive or True Masculine
• Selfish and needing to be right • Fearful of failure • Controlling and aggressive • Cold and distant • Extremely critical and judgemental • Stubborn, not in touch with emotions, argumentative	• Present without being distracted • Non-judgemental • Committed and powerful • Deep integrity and humbleness • Focus and discipline • Supportive and encouraging • Grounded and open to express vulnerabilities • Fair, logical and accountable
Negative or Wounded Feminine	**Positive or True Feminine**
• Low self-worth and insecure • Compromises integrity and values • Manipulative and jealous • Stuck in victimhood and negative self-talk • Excessively emotional and attached • Lacking intimacy and discipline • Afraid to speak the truth, lethargic • Struggles to set boundaries and people pleaser	• Sets boundaries • Loving, kind, nurturing and flexible • Vulnerable, compassionate and authentic • Receptive and confident of her body • Intuitive, creative and sensual • Assertive, fearless and secure • Emotionally mature • Inspiring and magnetic

The disparity in energy in both sexes is one of the main reasons for the lack of coherence in perceiving situations. Hence, identification becomes the key here. An excess of masculine energy can be balanced by grounding techniques in order to calm the aggressive and logical mind. Similarly, a surfeit of feminine energy can be balanced by turning inwards and creating a personal space, nurturing oneself away from packed schedules and long to-do lists.

EMERGENCE OF COEXISTENCE

'Equality is not a concept. It's not something we should be striving for. It's a necessity. Equality is like gravity, we need it to stand on this Earth as men and women...'

—JOSS WHEDON

Considering that men and women are born with distinct, inherent traits, it is puzzling why many men perceive themselves to be superior to women. The widespread belief in male superiority is thought to have originated from ancient tribes, where men were tasked with protecting women from being taken as valuable possessions during hostile invasions. Over the ages, this cultural practice of protecting women solidified the notion of women being the weaker sex. However, some biased individuals pushed the narrative of male superiority and confined women to domestic and reproductive roles.

This misguided perception of women as weak and in need of protection led to the rise of authoritarian regimes. During such times, women were confined to their homes, primarily for reproduction, and menstruation was associated with stigma. This societal pressure on women to solely bear children despite their capabilities and talents was unjust.

Centuries of patriarchy bred a desire for control, overshadowing the recognition of women's inherent wisdom. This dominance denied women choices in crucial aspects of life, be it menstrual, matrimony, childbirth, rest or self-expression. Unfortunately, patriarchy persists in modern society as well and women are subjected to inhumane treatment—forced marriages, sexual assaults and violence against women remain pressing issues. Both physical and verbal violence can leave deep scars on women's psyche and prevent them from fully participating in society. This must be addressed on a priority basis for an equal and healthy society.

Women continue to be objectified and seen as mere childbearing entities in many parts of our male-dominated society. It is not only men who perpetuate these biases but some women, including the elderly, unconsciously replicate the control and punishment they endured in their youth, perpetuating a cycle of mistreatment towards their daughters. Similarly, there are women who, driven by envy or a twisted sense of justice, have at times supported patriarchal systems, causing harm to fellow women, intentionally or unintentionally.

Unfortunately, as societal roles evolve within a dynamic environment, a discernible shift towards an ambiguous lifestyle emerges, fostering unhealthy behaviour. An ambiguous lifestyle implies a lack of clarity and structure in how individuals of both genders navigate their roles and responsibilities. This departure from the natural constitution of both genders not only leads to emotional health issues and strained relationships but also impacts overall well-being.

Today, women are constantly under pressure to uphold the 'superwoman' label, proving her mettle in all facets of life. These expectations have forced women to ignore their menstrual and emotional health in their struggle for self-reliance. They are quietly enduring health issues and masking their discomfort with painkillers, unaware of the potential harm being caused to their reproductive health.

By acknowledging the dualities and consciously integrating these binaries, individuals can cultivate greater clarity, abundance and harmonious relationships. Achieving balance for both genders involves open communication, equal partnership, respecting individuality and flexibility, prioritizing self-care and shared decision-making. This approach can lead to a life enriched with elevated experiences, improved work and transformative habits. A thriving and content relationship demands efforts from both parties, ensuring that each partner has profound love, unwavering respect and a steadfast commitment to equality in this shared journey through life.

INVOLVING MEN IN MENSTRUAL DISCUSSIONS

'When a man truly loves a woman
she becomes his weakness.
When a woman truly loves a man,
he becomes her strength.
This is called the exchange of power.'

—ANONYMOUS

Men's lack of understanding about the menstrual cycle is a direct result of the patriarchal system that deemed the topic taboo and failed to educate them. This foundational oversight has not only perpetuated gender bias but also hindered the development of healthy relationships between men and women. This ignorance is further compounded by the silent acquiescence of women who were conditioned to conceal their menstrual pain and discomfort. This conditioning is a significant reason why men feel uneasy when modern women openly express their menstrual struggles.

Men, as sons, brothers, fathers, cousins, colleagues, bosses, spouses and friends, have an integral part to play in the conversation related to menstruation. They must actively dispel the misconception that menstruation is solely a 'woman's issue'. Instead, the most valuable gift men can provide menstruating women around them is support and empathy. It's time for men to be educated about period pain being a natural biological occurrence. They must acknowledge that their existence is a result of their mothers' commitment to nature's assignment.

The true feminine can find its place in all its splendour only if we consciously dismantle the pressure of gender roles and stereotypes, ending the conflict with men and leading to a wholesome human coexistence and cooperation. By advancing through dialogues, discussions and awareness programmes, we can erase the damage of the past and make self-fulfilment a way of life. Society, at large, needs to comprehend that the pain of a man or woman needs to be seen in a humane manner.

Eckhart Tolle, a renowned author and spiritual teacher, eloquently emphasizes the potential of the yin/yang framework to foster heightened awareness of the delicate equilibrium within our society.[52] Cultivating an early awareness in children about coexistence, and interplay of their masculine and feminine attributes, lays the foundation for a nurturing society.

[52]Why Balancing Masculine and Feminine Energy is Essential | Yin and Yang with Eckhart Tolle, YouTube, https://www.youtube.com/watch?v=MIa-WABHOMY.

LIVING IN HARMONY

'Wherever you find a great man, you will find
a great mother or a great wife
standing behind him—or so they used to say.
It would be interesting to know how many great women
have had great fathers and husbands behind them.'

—DOROTHY L. SAYERS

Empowering women to occupy an equal position in society and at home is a crucial step towards creating a harmonious world. We must acknowledge and address the trauma women have endured at the hands of men and strive for equity by recognizing and valuing their voices in decision-making roles, particularly in matters of finance and governance. Women, too, must recognize that their achievements are the result of the support they receive from their families.

Throughout history, we've witnessed women ascending to positions of power and demonstrating remarkable competence. This accomplishment was made possible when certain men, recognizing talent, perseverance and resilience, willingly stepped aside, paving the way for women to lead and shine, showcasing their capabilities in steering significant initiatives and influencing positive change. This remarkable shift not only empowers women to lead but also illuminates the path for a more inclusive, diverse and collectively thriving future.

Nature, with its cyclical transformations, exemplifies the importance of surrendering power at the appropriate time for the sake of harmony. When both men and women allow each other to take centre stage, their relationships flourish in a harmonious coexistence.

I am delighted that the tide is slowly turning, resulting in a significant shift happening in the psyche of men, who are stakeholders and co-beneficiaries in the Universe. They are comprehending that they, too, stand to gain from healthy feminism.

Our dualities, previously misunderstood, undervalued, mocked at, threatened and feared, are now gradually being accepted in society and enabling humans to become well-rounded individuals.

THE BOTTOM LINE

Positions of power, ranging from grassroots levels to the highest ranks, are predominantly occupied by men. Therefore, as engineers, professors, health workers, teachers, family members, policymakers and bureaucrats, men have a pivotal role in introducing changes to eliminate gender disparity. With a rise in women's reproductive health issues and a prevailing disregard for menstruation, there's a pressing need for heightened awareness and empathy in workplaces, schools and universities. Let us work together to nurture a compassionate, equitable society where individuals are valued not for their gender but for their character.

NIMMI'S MANTRA

Real strength is in what makes us unique and different—not weaker or stronger but simply different.

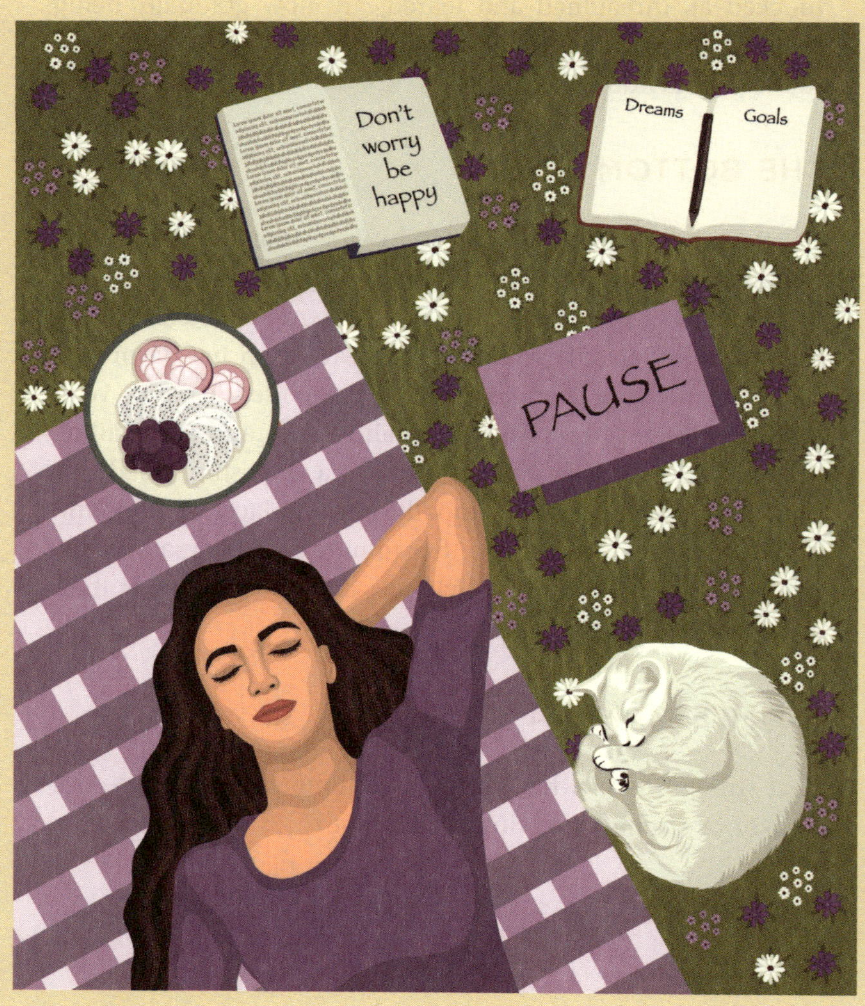

Don't worry be happy
Dreams
Goals
PAUSE

7
REPRODUCTIVE HEALTH

'Every human being is the author of his own health or disease.'

—GAUTAMA BUDDHA

When a woman attentively nurtures her 'red health' or menstrual well-being, her 'pink health', encompassing physical and mental well-being, is revitalized. I have coined these respective terms to signify how the menstrual cycle has a profound impact on a woman's physical and emotional health.[53] However, red health transcends menstruation; it embodies holistic wellness, embracing spiritual, physical and emotional efficacy. By prioritizing and caring for reproductive health, a woman can establish a robust foundation for her overall health and wellness.

COMMON CONCERNS

Menstruation is a natural biological occurrence; however, it can cause disruptions in a woman's daily activities if proper care is not taken. Some of the menstrual problems include an absence

[53]Rohatgi, Aishwarya, and Sambit Dash, 'Period Poverty and Mental Health of Menstruators during COVID-19 Pandemic: Lessons and Implications for the Future,' *Frontiers in Global Women's Health*, Vol. 4, 2023, 1128169, https://doi.org/10.3389/fgwh.2023.1128169.

of periods, irregular cycles, bleeding between periods, scanty or heavy flow, fertility issues, endometriosis, ovarian cysts and fibroids—all significant health concerns.

Menstrual health suffers greatly due to contraceptives, unplanned pregnancies, abortions, reproductive choices, sexually transmitted infections and unhealthy lifestyles. Further, psychological stressors such as ingrained beliefs, social pressures, gender discrimination and depression can impact menstrual health. Inconsistent periods or issues with red health often serve as the first indicators of extreme stress.

Hence, by adopting healthy lifestyle choices and consulting healthcare experts, we can treat the underlying causes and improve our menstrual (red) health.

Here are some common reproductive health concerns that every woman needs to be aware of:

Endometriosis

It is a condition in which the endometrial-like tissue grows outside the uterine cavity, on the ovaries, bowel and the tissues lining the pelvis. A possible factor is said to be retrograde menstruation.[54] Endometriosis is a chronic disease with extremely varied symptoms. It can cause blood clots, induce heavy bleeding, suppress the immune system and can also interfere with a woman's ability to conceive. Clinical studies indicate that endometriosis is a condition associated with high levels of chronic stress.[55]

Endometriosis manifests differently in each woman

---

[54] Mohamed, Abdul Wadood, 'Endometriosis', *Healthline*, Healthline Media, 12 January 2023, https://www.healthline.com/health/endometriosis.

[55] Reis, Fernando M., Larissa M. Coutinho, Silvia Vannuccini, Stefano Luisi, and Felice Petraglia, 'Is Stress a Cause or a Consequence of Endometriosis?', *Reproductive Sciences*, Vol. 27, 2020, 39–45, http://dx.doi.org/10.1007/s43032-019-00053-0.

and causes distressing symptoms. Menstrual pain can be excruciating and may persist throughout the month. Furthermore, this condition carries a burden of associated health challenges such as irritable bowel syndrome and infertility.[56] Endometriosis has a serious psychological and social impact on the lives of women, disturbing their sense of well-being and impeding professional growth.

Despite the severity of the pain, studies reveal that it can take 7–10 years for a woman to receive a diagnosis of endometriosis, indicating that many suffer in silence and may feel hesitant to seek help.[57]

Polycystic Ovarian Syndrome

Polycystic ovarian syndrome (PCOS) is considered to be the most prevalent menstrual disorder, affecting approximately 1 in 10 women of reproductive age worldwide. It is a medical condition characterized by the enlargement of the ovaries and is accompanied by the presence of small cysts along their outer edges. While the exact cause of PCOS remains unclear, it is believed to involve a combination of genetic factors as well as interactions between genes and the environment, which contributes to the development of this syndrome.[58]

PCOS can lead to various symptoms and health issues

[56]Eisenberg, Vered H., Dean H. Decter, Gabriel Chodick, Varda Shalev, and Clara Weil, 'Burden of Endometriosis: Infertility, Comorbidities, and Healthcare Resource Utilization', *Journal of Clinical Medicine*, Vol. 11, No. 4, 2022, 1133, https://doi.org/10.3390/jcm11041133.

[57]Frankel, Lexi R., 'A 10-Year Journey to Diagnosis with Endometriosis: An Autobiographical Case Report', *Cureus*, Vol. 14, No. 1, 2022, e21329, https://doi.org/10.7759/cureus.21329.

[58]'Polycystic Ovary Syndrome', *Office on Women's Health*, girlshealth.gov, 22 February 2021, https://www.womenshealth.gov/a-z-topics/polycystic-ovary-syndrome.

such as[59]:

Irregular menstrual cycles: Women with PCOS may experience irregular or infrequent periods or heavy bleeding.

Excess androgen hormones: Elevated levels of androgen, often referred to as 'male hormones' (though both men and women have them), can lead to symptoms like acne, hirsutism (excessive hair growth) and male-pattern baldness.

Ovulatory dysfunction: Many women with PCOS experience ovulatory dysfunction, which leads to difficulty in conceiving naturally. PCOS is one of the most common causes of infertility.

Polycystic ovaries: On ultrasound, the ovaries of individuals with PCOS may appear enlarged and contain small, fluid-filled sacs or cysts. However, not all individuals with PCOS have these cysts.

Metabolic issues: PCOS is often associated with metabolic disturbances such as insulin resistance, which can lead to weight gain, Type-2 diabetes and an increased risk of heart disease.

Other symptoms: PCOS can also be associated with a range of other symptoms, including mood disorders like depression and anxiety, sleep apnoea and irregular blood sugar levels, making it responsible for over 70% of ovarian issues.

PCOS significantly impacts the hormonal balance, and an unhealthy lifestyle, characterized by working at odd hours, prolonged periods of sitting, irregular sleep patterns, unhealthy dietary choices, leading a sedentary lifestyle, being overweight, undue exertion during menstruation and experiencing excessive

[59]'Polycystic Ovary Syndrome', *World Health Organization*, https://www.who.int/news-room/fact-sheets/detail/polycystic-ovary-syndrome.

fear or grief, can further aggravate symptoms (vata imbalance). If not diagnosed and treated early, it can cause complications later on in life.

Uterine Fibroids

While the cause of uterine fibroids is unknown, excess oestrogen has been linked to the formation of these fibroids, which erupt as non-cancerous growths in or on the wall of the uterus. Oestrogen and progesterone reach peak levels during a woman's reproductive years, which leads to the development of fibroids. Over 80% of the female population experiences fibroids at some point in their lives and data indicates that genetics, obesity and a sedentary lifestyle are the primary risk factors.[60]

Women who experience menarche at an early age are considered more susceptible to this medical condition. These fibroids are hormone-dependent and cause erratic symptoms, such as heaviness in the lower abdomen, sudden gushing of blood during periods, pelvic pain, lack of ovulation, abnormal weight gain (indicative of kapha imbalance in Ayurvedic medicine) and infertility.

Amenorrhea

Amenorrhea is defined as the absence of periods during the reproductive years of a woman's life and can occur either due to genetic conditions or malnutrition. It can also be caused by excessive weight loss, eating disorders, strenuous exercise, substance abuse or side effects of certain long-term medications.[61]

[60]'Fibroids,' *The John Hopkins University*, https://www.hopkinsmedicine.org/health/conditions-and-diseases/uterine-fibroids.

[61]Nawaz, Gul, and Alan D. Rogol, 'Amenorrhea,' *National Library of Medicine*, 12 June 2023, https://www.ncbi.nlm.nih.gov/books/NBK482168/.

Menorrhagia

Menorrhagia is a common disorder, which refers to heavy and prolonged bleeding that lasts over a week, along with other symptoms such as severe abdominal pain and dizziness. The main causes of menorrhagia are uterine fibroids, thyroid dysfunction, hormonal imbalance and blood clotting issues, which can lead to anaemia and sometimes cervical cancer.[62] If not treated early, this medical condition can interfere with the normal routine of daily life.

Oligomenorrhea

This disorder of extremely minimal bleeding and infrequent periods can occur due to multiple reasons, such as fluctuating hormone levels, thyroid issues, obesity, female genital tuberculosis and extreme weight loss/gain.[63]

Dysmenorrhea

Dysmenorrhea is the medical term for persistent menstrual cramps. It can manifest as throbbing or cramping pain or discomfort in the lower abdomen and pelvis before or during menstruation. Its most common symptoms are nausea, vomiting, giddiness and diarrhoea. Dysmenorrhea can significantly impact a person's quality of life and is caused by uterine fibroids or other medical conditions.[64]

---

[62] Braun, Ashley, 'Heavy Menstrual Bleeding (Menorrhagia)', *Verywell Health*, Dotdash Media, Inc., 24 October 2023, https://www.verywellhealth.com/heavy-menstrual-bleeding-menorrhagia-5224454.

[63] Heitz, David, 'Oligomenorrhea', *Healthline*, Healthline Media, 9 July 2017, https://www.healthline.com/health/oligomenorrhea.

[64] 'Dysmenorrhea', *The John Hopkins University*, https://www.hopkinsmedicine.org/health/conditions-and-diseases/dysmenorrhea.

Infertility

There has been a surge in the number of women grappling with infertility issues. Infertility is a result of other underlying medical conditions such as PCOS, uterine fibroids, endometriosis, pelvic inflammatory disease (which may lead to scarring, resulting in blockages in fallopian tubes) and primary ovarian insufficiency.[65]

Infertility is rapidly emerging as a prominent concern among women, serving as a stark reflection of the stress and challenges they navigate while juggling demanding careers (often involving prolonged periods of sitting and irregular working hours), managing households, sustaining relationships and dealing with limited emotional and financial support. Moreover, the increase in the usage of electronics has also raised questions about its potential impact on fertility and other health issues.[66]

HEALTHY VAGINA, HEALTHY YOU

Vaginal health is a crucial component of a woman's overall health, which affects fertility, desire for intimacy and self-confidence. Neglecting menstrual hygiene can have a negative impact on vaginal health and consequently affect reproductive health in the long term.[67]

Poor menstrual hygiene can lead to unpleasant and

---

[65]'What Are Some Possible Causes of Female Infertility?,' *National Institute of Child Health and Human Development*, 31 January 2017, https://www.nichd.nih.gov/health/topics/infertility/conditioninfo/causes/causes-female.

[66]Kundu, Sampurna, Balhasan Ali, and Preeti Dhillon, 'Surging Trends of Infertility and Its Behavioural Determinants in India,' *PLoS One*, Vol. 18, No. 7, 2023, e0289096, https://doi.org/10.1371/journal.pone.0289096.

[67]'The Connection Between Menstrual Hygiene and Vaginal Health,' *Gynin*, https://www.gynin.com/blog/the-connection-between-menstrual-hygiene-and-vaginal-health/.

potentially harmful consequences for menstruating women. The prolonged retention of menstrual blood in pads, cups or cloth can foster the growth of bacteria, leading to infections and unpleasant odours. In some cases, this can cause rashes, itching and inflammation. To maintain proper hygiene and avoid these issues, it is necessary to regularly replace soiled pads or cloth and keep the vaginal area clean and dry.

Among the various indicators of vaginal health is the colour of your vaginal discharge, which is a fluid that exits our bodies through the vaginal opening.[68] This discharge is a mixture of cells and bacteria that lubricates and protects the vagina. It is a natural process, resulting in a clear, white or off-white fluid, unless it has an unusual consistency, colour or odour.

White discharge is generally an indication of the approaching period and occurs soon after ovulation during the luteal stage. Discharge may either be thin and abundant around the time of ovulation or slightly thick and more opaque at other times, depending on one's menstrual cycle and body type. Progesterone, which is at its peak during the initial luteal phase, is the reason for this milky discharge. It is nature's way of ensuring a smooth and easy process for intercourse and conception. Hence, it is a sign of good fertility for those planning for a child.

However, when the discharge is dark yellow in colour and is accompanied by itching, pain, increase in volume, foul odour or burning sensations, it may indicate fungal or bacterial infections. You should visit a medical professional in case of such abnormal discharges.

---

[68]Galan, Nicole, 'A Color-coded Guide to Vaginal Discharge', *Medical News Today*, Healthline Media, 22 December 2023, https://www.medicalnewstoday.com/articles/321131.

There is a pressing need for comprehensive support for and understanding of women's reproductive health, as its complications need immediate medical intervention. Additionally, women should concentrate on maintaining a consistent sleep schedule, eating nutritiously and alleviating stress by engaging in meaningful hobbies, yoga and various forms of physical exercise. It is vital to keep track of your menstrual cycle and note abnormal symptoms such as heavy bleeding, spotting, intense cramping, large blood clots and painful bowel movements—these significant symptoms need regular monitoring and medical help.

It helps us to keep abreast of any changes that may happen within our bodies, which can result in early detection of abnormalities, saving us from major reproductive diseases.

FOCUS ON HABITS, NOT HORMONES

When facing health issues, it is important to introspect and ask ourselves these questions: Are we prepared to slow down to nurture ourselves? Are we open to lifestyle changes?

The truth is that women's lives and bodily functions are largely governed by two sex hormones: oestrogen and progesterone.[69] Many women suffer from underlying health conditions that negatively impact these hormone levels, leading to menstrual irregularities. This can be managed if symptoms are identified and addressed promptly, preventing even more severe complications.

Here are some positive lifestyle changes we can incorporate into our lives.

[69] Gorvett, Zaria, 'How the Menstrual Cycle Changes Women's Brains—For Better,' *BBC Future*, 7 August 2018, https://www.bbc.com/future/article/20180806-how-the-menstrual-cycle-changes-womens-brains-every-month.

Lifestyle: Life is a long lesson in humility. By consciously removing the extreme contrasts of neither being 'superhuman' nor remaining 'sedentary', amending irregular eating habits and reducing working at odd hours, we can prevent health disruptions. It would do well to keep in mind that excessive use of electronic devices and over-exercising are all capable of messing with our hormones.

Sleep deprivation: Sleep is a panacea for most physical and mental ailments. But sadly it is also the most underrated aspect of life. Sleep deprivation is known to raise cortisol levels, reduce glucose tolerance and amplify sympathetic nervous system activity, thereby increasing stress and overstimulating the hormones.[70]

Self-medication: Modernization has brought the world to our fingertips through the Internet. The accessibility of information online leads many to self-diagnose and self-treat with painkillers, pills, and other drugs without a proper medical consultation, which can create a surfeit of toxins within the body.

Beauty products: We live in an era in which beauty rules over health consciousness. The liberal use of synthesized and chemical-laden beauty products, which have flooded the markets, contaminates the body with toxins, making the need to take the natural (alternative) route more urgent than ever.

Diet choices: Women, especially young girls, need a nutritional diet, and not a fad diet that promises dramatic results. Media and societal pressures push them towards a certain body

---

[70] Hirotsu, Camila, Sergio Tufik, and Monica Levy Andersen, 'Interactions Between Sleep, Stress, and Metabolism: From Physiological to Pathological Conditions', *Sleep Science*, Vol. 8, No. 3, 2015, 143–152, https://doi.org/10.1016/j.slsci.2015.09.002.

image, which has led to faulty dieting and eating disorders. Additionally, processed foods and artificial flavours are significant contributors to various health issues.

Environment: Issues such as soil degradation, pollution, landfills and climate change and its effects on the oceans, rivers and lakes may seem to be beyond our control. However, this deterioration in air quality and chemical infiltration has indirectly impacted women's menstrual health. Opting for sustainable, green menstrual products is a small step towards the mitigation of climate change.

Social factors: Emotional and social issues such as gender discrimination, patriarchy and reluctance to discuss menstrual problems result in suppressed emotions, leading to hormone fluctuations. Creating awareness is a prime necessity and the only solution to this problem.

Addictions: Addiction, in any form, be it substance or behaviour-based, has the power to wreak havoc on an individual's physical, mental and social well-being. From alcohol, drugs and coffee to binge eating, excessive sleeping, compulsive shopping, unnecessary plastic surgeries and even the use of birth control pills, the compulsion to escape reality often stems from mental health issues and can result in serious health problems. Birth control pills, in particular, contain synthetic oestrogen that can alter the natural menstrual cycle and disrupt reproductive health.[71] There are no shortcuts to good health and it is imperative to break away from unhealthy dependencies to live a healthy life. By treating the underlying causes of addiction

[71] Kennedy, Madeline, 'How Birth Control Pills Work by Tricking the Body into Thinking It's Already Pregnant', *Business Insider*, Insider Inc, 23 May 2020, https://www.businessinsider.com/guides/health/reproductive-health/how-does-birth-control-work?IR=T.

and mental health struggles, one can restore the balance of their reproductive system, enhancing overall life quality.

A GIFT TO OURSELVES

One small step towards preventive measures can become a giant leap away from diseases. Periodic gynaecological examinations, pap smear tests and ultrasonography of the pelvis are crucial for identifying potential uterine issues. Consultations with registered medical practitioners can enlighten us about our bodies' responses to our lifestyles, making treatments more efficient.

Individual approach: Every woman is physiologically unique because of her bodily constitution or doshas (vata, pitta and kapha). She needs to move in harmony with nature and weigh the benefits of holistic treatments against the long-term side effects of drugs. If each woman consciously addresses her reproductive problems by prioritizing self-care and adopting a personalized programme, she can enjoy 'positive periods' and live a fulfilling life.

In his book *Dr Mathai's Holistic Health Guide for Women,* Dr Isaac Mathai empowers women to take charge of their well-being through holistic means.[72] This visionary healer underscores the importance of prioritizing reproductive health and utilizing alternative methods such as Ayurvedic *panchakarma* treatments, homoeopathy, naturopathy as well as complimentary therapies such as yoga, acupressure, reflexology and Chinese acupuncture. He also encourages making simple DIY home remedies to address the underlying cause of any disease or hormonal imbalance that helps in reducing inflammation.

The renowned healer also emphasizes the use of gentle

[72]Mathai, Isaac, *Dr Mathai's Holistic Health Guide for Women*, Random House, Inc., New York City, NY, 1 January 2013.

naturopathic treatments such as mud baths, hip baths, herbal steam baths, T-packs and hot compresses to the abdomen as adjuncts to conventional treatments for reducing inflammation, stabilizing hormones and stimulating blood flow to the uterus. These remedies can induce normal menstrual bleeding. He asserts that while conventional medicine takes care of the body, alternative therapies attend to the mind, leading to wholesome living.

Dr Mathai advocates for personalized treatments, taking into account the individual's medical history, age, body constitution and emotional health. He emphasizes the importance of tracking nutrition, functional variations, chronic illnesses, stress levels, daily habits and potential impacts of being on long-term medication for optimal results.

THE BOTTOM LINE

A healthy reproductive system is not only the absence of disease but also a state of overall well-being. The right foundation laid during adolescence to prioritize reproductive health by endorsing education, menstrual awareness, meaningful rituals, nutrition and holistic practices enables every woman to lead a healthy life and achieve harmony in all aspects of her existence.

NIMMI'S MANTRA

Provide nurturing care for your womb for optimal health.

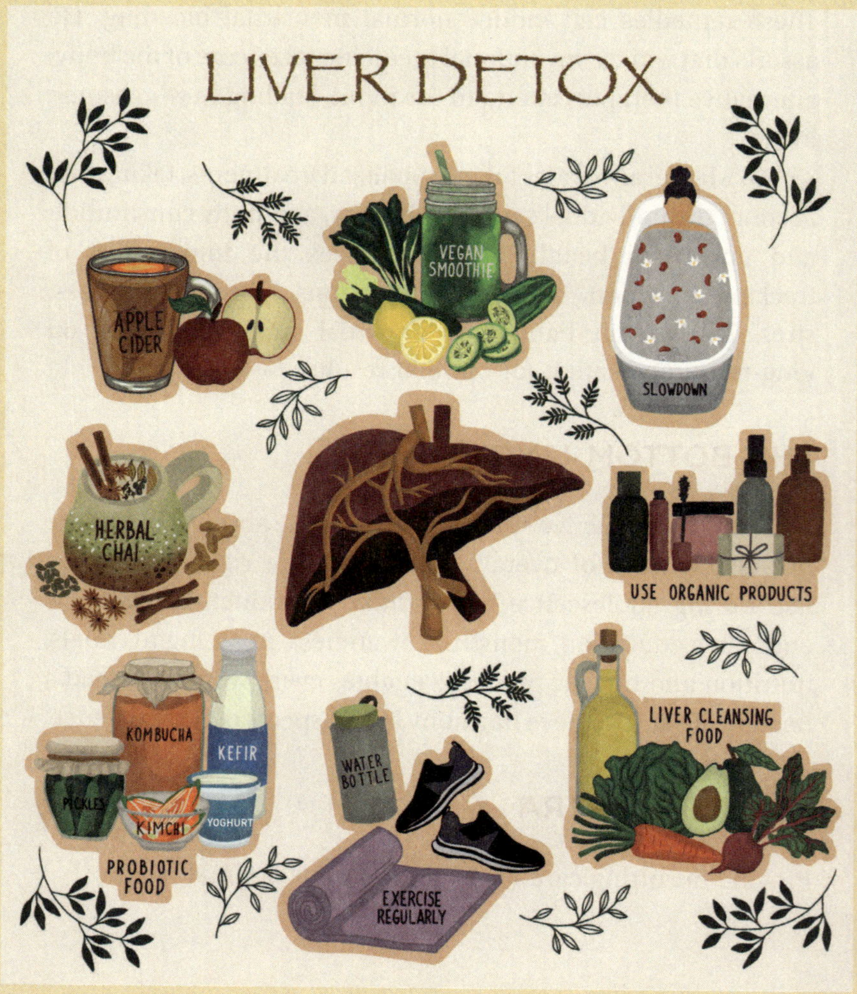
LIVER DETOX
APPLE CIDER
VEGAN SMOOTHIE
SLOWDOWN
HERBAL CHAI
USE ORGANIC PRODUCTS
KOMBUCHA
KEFIR
PICKLES
KIMCHI
YOGHURT
PROBIOTIC FOOD
WATER BOTTLE
EXERCISE REGULARLY
LIVER CLEANSING FOOD

8

THE LIVER EFFECT

'Our entire personality, our energy level and how we cope is hormonal.'

—SANDRA TSING LOH

Hormones, the master controller of metabolism, exert a significant influence on various bodily functions. These chemical messengers circulate within the bloodstream and any disruption in their functions can profoundly impact mood, metabolism, appetite and reproductive health.

The menstrual cycle operates under the guidance of various glands and hormones. These hormonal activities are managed by signals emanating from the brain. Central to this regulation are the interactions between LH, FSH and female sexual hormones, which wield considerable influence over menstrual cycles, fertility and pregnancy. Moreover, these hormones affect a woman's body weight, hair growth, bone density and muscle development.

This chapter will explore the workings of the female sex hormones (oestrogen and progesterone) and explain why keeping them balanced should be a priority.

Oestrogen Dominance

Oestrogen, often referred to as the reigning monarch of menstruation, plays a pivotal role during puberty in adolescent girls. Oestrogen is also known as a 'happy hormone'[73]; as it slows down the ageing process, plumps the skin, enhances digestion and boosts serotonin levels for better sleep. In addition to regulating the menstrual cycle, it ensures the smooth functioning of the cognitive, musculoskeletal and cardiovascular systems of the body.

If both oestrogen and its counterpart, progesterone, maintain a rhythmic cycle, they are immensely beneficial not just for menstrual health but also for our cognitive well-being. Any imbalances in these two hormones, which may occur at different periods of the menstrual cycle, results in our bodies facing a plethora of health-related challenges.

Although both men and women struggle due to hormonal imbalances, women suffer significantly more because of oestrogen dominance. Oestrogen levels rise and fall during each menstrual cycle. Its dominance is related to progesterone deficiency in women,[74] which can cause mood swings, fatigue, distorted sleep, unusual weight gain, change in bleeding patterns and even infertility.

This imbalance in the oestrogen-progesterone ratio increases the risk of breast cancer, PCOS, endometriosis, fibrocystic breasts, thyroid, breast tenderness, decreased sex drive, obesity, skin discolouration, temporary hair loss, increased cortisol and brain fog. Most of the symptoms associated with menstruation, such as heavy and prolonged periods with clotting, sluggishness and feelings of depression and anxiety, are also due to oestrogen dominance.

---

[73]Biali, Susan, '5 Happy Hormones and How to Boost Them Naturally,' *Best Health*, Reader's Digest Magazines Ltd., https://www.besthealthmag.ca/article/how-to-boost-your-happy-hormones/.

[74]Mahannah, Kathleen, '10 Signs You May Have Estrogen Dominance,' *Dr. Kathleen Mahannah, ND*, 18 November 2020, https://drkathleenmahannah.com/blog/estrogen-dominance.

Oestrogen's Influence on Liver

Oestrogen shares an exceptional bond with the liver. While the body is dependent on the liver for various vital functions, the organ itself relies on oestrogen for its optimal functioning. Therefore, a balanced oestrogen is crucial for the liver to function normally.[75]

The liver, a major metabolic organ, converts the nutrients in our food into substances that the body can utilize. It also filters and eliminates harmful toxins and surplus hormones from the bloodstream. However, its relentless efforts can be burdened by unhealthy diets, consumption of alcohol and synthetic cola, sleep deprivation, stress, long-term medication use, environmental pollution, and exposure to plastics and endocrine-disrupting skincare and cleansing products.

If filtration is impaired, the liver fails to eliminate excess oestrogen, leading to its reabsorption into the bloodstream, which may result in weight gain, bloating and ovarian cysts. Fibre-rich and plant-based diets may help reduce oestrogen levels and maintain healthy oestrogen levels, respectively.

In her book *It's Not My Head, It's My Hormones*, Dr Marion Gluck offers insightful advice on taming erratic hormones and living a healthy life. She also discusses how to make your hormones your allies by optimizing your menstrual, mental and physical health.[76]

To navigate hormonal shifts it is crucial for women:

- to recognize that oestrogen production dominates during the first half of the menstrual cycle while progesterone production is higher in the second half.

[75]'How to Optimize Liver Function to Rebalance Hormones in Women', *Hormones & Balance*, 3 September 2013, https://hormonesbalance.com/articles/the-role-of-the-liver-in-female-hormone-balance/.

[76]Gluck, Marion, *It's Not My Head, It's My Hormones*, Orion Spring, London, 28 November 2019.

- to understand that our bodies can produce more progesterone only after ovulation occurs.
- to be aware that if ovulation does not occur for unknown reasons, one may encounter hormonal imbalances and fertility problems. Symptoms such as irregular cycles, pain, PMS, bloating and heavy bleeding are signals through which our bodies attempt to alert us to take charge of our valuable health.

Influence of Progesterone

Progesterone is known for its calming effects on both the mind and body and is hence classified as a neurosteroid.[77] It stimulates the brain's gamma-aminobutyric acid or GABA receptors, which are associated with feelings of well-being and tranquillity. It helps regulate body weight during menstruation and contributes to a sense of happiness. Its primary functions include regulating the menstrual cycle and preventing the overgrowth of certain types of cancerous cells in the endometrial lining. Stress hormones, thyroid imbalance, menstrual irregularities, miscarriages or menopause can affect progesterone production and lead to conditions such as depression, anxiety and infertility in women.

As progesterone responds strongly to stress and anxiety, addressing these deep-rooted issues can give better results than focusing solely on symptoms. A simple blood test, taken one week before periods, can detect its levels. We can bring positive changes to our lifestyles and follow healthy habits, such as consuming a balanced diet and getting regular exercise, to strengthen the liver's natural detoxification process, thereby prompting a healthy menstruation.

---

[77] Christiansen, Sherry, 'How Progesterone Promotes Brain Health,' *Verywell Health*, Dotdash Media, Inc., 15 September 2021, https://www.verywellhealth.com/progesterone-and-brain-health-4589255.

The human body is a sophisticated machine that needs regular maintenance. Connect with a professional medical practitioner and get your hormone levels checked, especially the levels of estrone (E1), estradiol (E2) and estriol (E3) (the three major types of oestrogen in women) in the blood, also known as oestrogenic hormone tests, before devising any personalized treatment plan.[78]

XENOESTROGENS

Women need to be aware of a modern-day poison called xenoestrogens that can invade and take root in all aspects of their lives. Knowledge of how these endocrine-disrupting chemicals can negatively manipulate the hormonal process is a step towards better health.

Xenoestrogens—also known as environmental oestrogens—are harmful chemicals found in everyday household items such as cosmetics, hair dyes, fabric softeners, genetically modified food, plastic containers in the kitchen, contaminated water and even in the air.[79] They are also present in livestock and agrochemical industrial products. These can also be found in food products, which can be injected with synthetic hormones, including dairy, animal products, commercially raised meat, chicken, beef, pork, ice cream, animal fats and vegetable oils (and corn and soy too).

These chemicals enter the human body by mimicking the functions of naturally produced oestrogen, sending incorrect signals to the brain and blocking the natural receptors. This can be seriously detrimental, especially to hormone-sensitive

[78] WebMD Editorial Contributors, 'Estrogen Test', *WebMD*, 9 September 2022, https://www.webmd.com/women/estrogen-test.

[79] Velasco, Melissa, 'Your Home Needs A Detox!', *Eighty-Six the Endo*, 21 November 2021, https://eightysixtheendo.com/detox-environmental-estrogens/.

organs such as the breasts, uterus and immune and neurological systems. These invisible chemicals can prove harmful if they enter into the body's tissues and cells, bypassing liver filtration. The widespread use of these toxic chemicals in everyday products is concerning, highlighting the urgent need to reduce exposure by advocating for organic and natural alternatives for our health.

Understanding the roles of both oestrogen and progesterone hormones is extremely important as an imbalance in one hormone can negatively affect the other and cause quite an upheaval within the body.

SECRETS TO A HEALTHY LIVER

Every human body possesses a powerful innate detoxification system. The liver, being the primary filter, cleanses and purifies the blood by preventing pathogens from passing into the bloodstream and eliminating them from the body through sweat, saliva and urine. Enhancing liver function can be achieved by incorporating fibre-rich food into our daily diet, supporting natural detoxification. Consuming food that aids the elimination process would be the best way to maintain a healthy liver.

Here are some steps that can be incorporated into our daily routines for healthy liver functioning:

Step 1: Minimize or Avoid Liver Damage

Reset your hormones with fibre-rich vegetables, greens and fruits to balance your oestrogen.

- Keep track of all the symptoms caused by oestrogen dominance and minimize exposure to them.
- Limit the use of plastics.

- Opt for natural/herbal pesticides and home-cleaning products.
- Check for fluoride content in the water supply and toothpaste and avoid or reduce its usage.
- Replace non-stick cookware or conventional steel with safer alternatives, such as ceramic, food-grade stainless steel or cast iron.
- Use copper, silver or wooden utensils, as they increase the energy or life of food.
- Choose paraben-free options in products such as shampoos, lotions or soaps.
- Learn to identify the list of ingredients before buying packaged food.
- Avoid artificial sweeteners; fried, canned, factory-made, processed or refined foods; white bread; genetically modified grains and vegetables; and also some of the nightshade vegetables as they are challenging for the liver to process.
- Choose grass-fed, ethically-raised animal protein; free-range eggs; and A2 milk, ghee and yoghurt.
- Avoid processed meat and dairy products from factory-raised animals that are laden with artificial hormones.
- Consume healthy fats, such as extra virgin coconut oil, sesame oil, olive oil and medium-chain triglyceride or MCT oil.
- Address any food allergies and intolerances by keeping a note of their underlying symptoms.
- Consume more organic-certified and locally produced fruits, cruciferous vegetables, beets, garlic, ginger, lemon and other liver-friendly vegetables. If possible grow your own safe food in your backyard or kitchen.
- Include herbs such as *shatavari*, neem and ashwagandha to balance hormones.
- Say no to illicit drugs and smoking and limit or avoid consumption of alcohol.

- Avoid birth control pills unless prescribed otherwise.
- Monitor thyroid levels by regularly undertaking T3 or T4 tests.
- Massage the pressure point (or the tendon) between the big toe and the second toe, as the nerves present here are directly connected to the liver (acupressure massage).
- Address mental stress issues by seeking professional help.
- Take a 15-minute nap to refresh.
- Maintain healthy body weight by walking, stretching and exercising regularly.

Women experiencing significant menstrual health issues should consider eliminating inappropriate diet combinations from their routines.

Step 2: Detoxify through Vegetable Smoothies and Concoctions

Build a simple detox programme for each morning, which may start after you consume plain or lukewarm water. Consider the following options:

- Have a spoonful of lemon juice or apple cider vinegar (rich in Vitamin C) with honey and warm water. This can help balance the body's PH levels.
- Steep half a lemon with its rind and a 1″ piece of ginger or 1/4 tsp ginger powder together in a cup of boiled water. Stir and strain the concoction before drinking.
- Enjoy vegetable smoothies that help nourish and purify the liver. Harness the benefits of succulent ingredients like beetroot, carrots, cucumber, kale, spinach, coriander, mint, Indian ash gourd and bottle gourd. To create your own liver-friendly smoothies, it is essential to learn and understand the nature of various herbs and vegetables. Observe how your body constitution (vata, pitta or kapha; detailed in Chapter

9) reacts to different combinations of smoothies mentioned above. This experimentation will help you customize your smoothies to your specific needs.

Embrace this morning ritual for greater well-being, savouring each sip and chewing the fibrous pulp to unleash the full potency of enzymes to kick-start the digestive process.

It is recommended to seek the guidance of a qualified nutritionist or alternative therapist before considering these options, especially if you have a medical condition like high blood pressure and imbalances in sodium or potassium levels, to avoid adverse effects on your health.

Step 3: Fasting

'Fasting is the first principle of medicine;
fast and see the strength of the spirit reveal itself.'

—RUMI

Discussions on detoxification will never be complete without a foray into fasting as it allows the body to cleanse itself naturally.

According to ancient Indian scriptures, fasting on occasions such as *Ekadashi* (Hindu fasting ritual) and following the movements of the Moon have a direct correlation with the mind. Through mindful abstinence, this sacred act grants a well-deserved respite to the internal organs and rejuvenates the digestive system by purging toxic substances.

Science has confirmed the plethora of benefits of intermittent fasting, including regulation of blood glucose levels, decreased risk of heart disease and cancer, protection against autoimmune diseases, cell regeneration, weight loss, enhanced sleep and optimal menstrual health via hormonal balance.[80] This powerful practice is crucial for those who consume meat-heavy diet and also for sedentary vegetarians who regularly consume oil-laden, fatty, sugary and creamy foods. Fasting is the most humbling way of offering gratitude to the Universe and a means of seeking spiritual abundance.

Fasting Tips for Different Cycles

Amy Shah, M.D., an integrative medicine doctor with training from Cornell, Columbia and Harvard Universities, shares her expertise on how a woman's hormonal landscape changes exponentially throughout her monthly cycle.[81] She says that every woman requires a personalized fitness regime that will work in harmony with fasting.

Shah suggests beginning with a short fast during the initial days of menstruation and gradually increasing the fasting hours as hormones rise in the follicular phase. She recommends extending the fasting hours during ovulation for cleansing and detoxification to stabilize hormonal fluctuations. She also advises against fasting or suggests reducing fasting hours considerably during the luteal phase when the body is at its most vulnerable.

In her book *I'm So Effing Tired,* Shah recommends reducing activities one is habitually used to, during the luteal phase, that may exacerbate PMS symptoms and irregular bleeding patterns.[82] Shah notes that even those who are on a hormonal pill might not experience recognizable changes in their mood

[80]Suchitra, M.R., and S. Parthasarathy, 'Intermittent Fasting on the Ekadashi Day and the Role of Spiritual Nutrition', *Current Research in Nutrition and Food Science*, Vol. 9, No. 1, 2021, 122–126, http://dx.doi.org/10.12944/CRNFSJ.9.1.12.

[81]'How To Fast and Eat During Your Menstrual Cycle', Dr. Amy Shah MD, 21 January 2022, https://amymdwellness.com/blogs/news/how-to-fast-and-eat-during-your-menstrual-cycle.

[82]Shah, Amy, *I'm So Effing Tired: A Proven Plan to Beat Burnout, Boost Your Energy, and Reclaim Your Life*, Mariner Books, Boston, MA, 2 March 2021.

and energy levels but still should be mindful of fasting in all menstrual cycles, and check if they're feeling fatigued or stressed. She underscores the importance of understanding the rhythm of the menstrual cycles to adopt a flexible fasting schedule.

Keeping these recommendations in mind, women must monitor how their bodies react by restricting certain foods during intermittent fasting. The female body, unlike the male body, is sensitive to major shifts in calorie restrictions. Further, indiscriminate fasting can disrupt the flow of hormones, running the risk of irregular periods, infertility and other health issues. Hence women should consider a modified approach, opting for regular, short-term fasts, and be cautious of calorie deficits to avoid adverse effects.

Fasting is both a science and a meaningful ritual but it should be practised under professional guidance. Mindful fasting can be incredibly useful for optimizing productivity, achieving and maintaining a healthy weight, fertility, libido, energy and mood.

As Plutarch wisely said, 'Instead of using medicine, rather, fast [for] a day.'[83] Investing in our health, whether in the form of time, money or energy, is essential. Mindful fasting can be considered a cure for certain ailments, beyond merely a weight loss strategy.[84] It improves cognitive function and stalls age-related cognitive decline.

THE BOTTOM LINE

The hormonal cycle may be the reason for many of our woes but it is also a victim of our maltreatment. Habits such as eating

[83]'Fasting and Purification,' *Greek Medicine*, David K. Osborn L. Ac., http://www.greekmedicine.net/hygiene/Fasting_and_Purification.html.

[84]Phillips, Matthew C.L., 'Fasting as a Therapy in Neurological Disease,' *Nutrients*, Vol. 11, No. 10, 2019, 2501, https://doi.org/10.3390/nu11102501.

nutrient-dense food, fasting mindfully, finding the right balance between work and rest, ensuring quality sleep, adhering to a regular exercise and meditation regime, and importantly, finding fulfilment in productivity can bring down stress levels and keep your hormones happy, healthy and in harmony.

NIMMI'S MANTRA

Your body possesses the innate ability to heal itself; it is your mind that you have to convince.

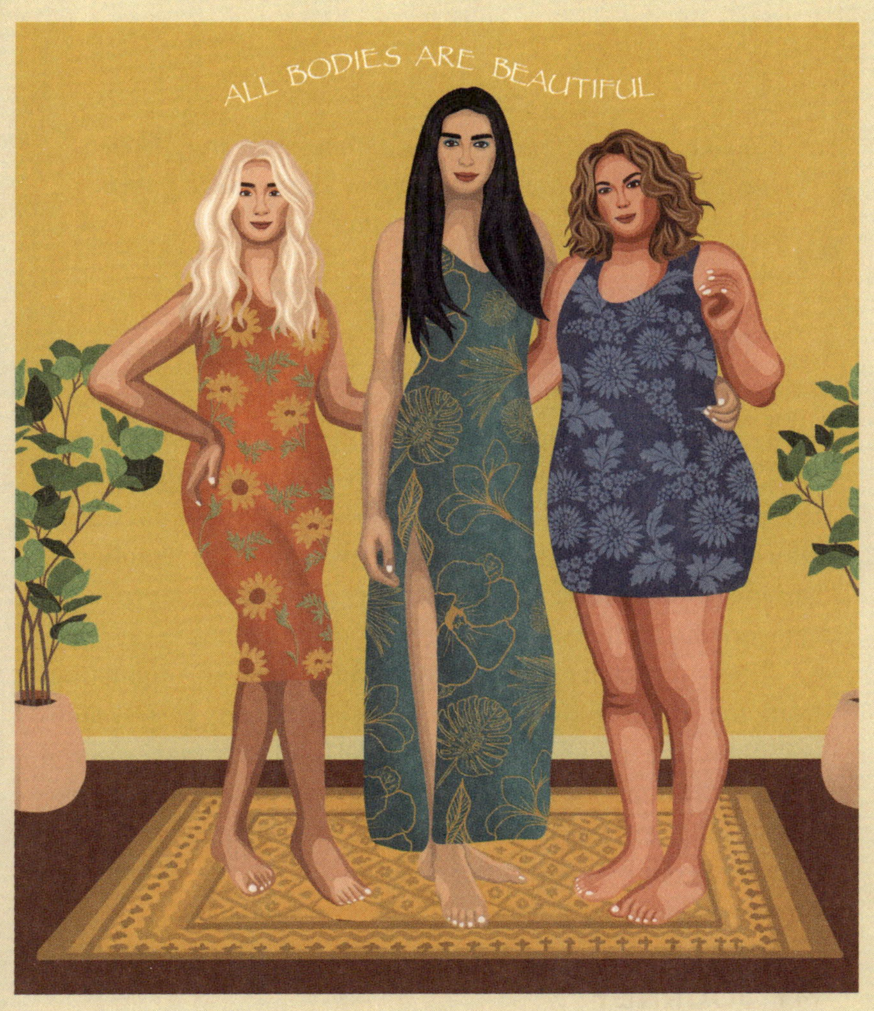
ALL BODIES ARE BEAUTIFUL

9

KNOW YOUR TRIDOSHAS

'If your body and mind were a handwritten story, then vata is the ink, pitta is the pen and kapha is the paper. Each one is vital.'

—ANONYMOUS

The human body is unique and complex; it is not a 'one size fits all' proposition. This is the fundamental concept behind Ayurveda philosophy, which recognizes that individuals may have a slender, average or robust physique, which may be attributed to both physical and emotional variances. Ayurveda acknowledges these differences by categorizing them as body constitutions or doshas.

These principles are timeless and universal, originating from the Vedic tradition of holistic healthcare. This system combines the physical, psychological and spiritual aspects of an individual, focusing on treating and healing the whole body. Aptly termed 'the knowledge of life,' Ayurveda aims to rejuvenate our bodies by addressing the root cause of illnesses through holistic wellness.

MY JOURNEY

Embarking on a transformative journey in my early twenties, I found solace and wisdom in the holistic approach of Ayurvedic philosophy. Immersing myself in the cornerstone works of esteemed Ayurvedic luminaries such as Vasant Lad and David Frawley, along with insights from the yogis of the Bihar School of Yoga, I delved deep into the ancient system of medicine to discern my unique dosha type. This exploration into Ayurveda offered me profound insights into self-awareness and fostered a harmonious connection with my distinctive bodily constitution, empowering me to celebrate life's richness with newfound appreciation.

Below, I offer a distilled essence of Ayurvedic wisdom, aimed at guiding you to uncover your dosha. This endeavour aims to shed light on recognizing and leveraging your strengths while addressing vulnerabilities, guiding you towards holistic well-being and self-discovery.

UNDERSTANDING YOUR TRIDOSHAS

Vata, pitta and kapha are the tridoshas (three body types) of Ayurveda and are classified under the term doshas or constitution, which translates to prakriti (our true nature) in Sanskrit. This chapter will focus on these doshas, exploring how they form our unique body types, with distinct physiological and psychological tendencies that remain with us throughout our lives, serving as the genetic blueprint for our well-being.

To begin with, we need to understand that prakriti/dosha is inherited while *vikruti* represents the imbalance of doshas arising from the environment one inhabits as well as the present state of body and mind. For instance, acquired habits like unhealthy eating, sleeping patterns and prejudice are all irregularities that lead to emotional imbalance. Therefore, identifying vikruti imbalances with the assistance of qualified Ayurvedic practitioners becomes crucial. They take into account a person's age, geographical location, occupation and life goals, and may recommend Ayurvedic panchakarma treatment or other personalized healing programs to balance vikruti dosha.

Acknowledging and respecting individual prakriti and vikruti in all four phases of the menstrual cycle can help us to address hormonal variations and navigate our lives with ease and confidence.[85] The knowledge of our true nature makes it easy for us to plan necessary dietary and lifestyle changes, along with choosing the suitable professions, hobbies and activities, offering an insight into building mental resilience to enhance the quality of life.

DETERMINING OUR INDIVIDUALITY

Ayurveda recognizes five elemental forces—air, water, fire, ether and earth (*pancha bhutas* or *tattvas*)—as the foundation of life. Ayurvedic philosophy specifically implies that man and earth are composed of these elements, albeit in varying combinations and ratios. These elements circulate as cosmic intelligence or as subtle energies in the body and mind.

These elements combine to form the doshas or bio-energies, which influence various aspects of life, including physiology, health, behaviour and relationships. The three primary doshas are vata, pitta and kapha, which are respectively correlated to ectomorph, mesomorph and endomorph body types in conventional science.

It is common for any individual to have one or two of the doshas dominating over the other, which becomes the determining factor for any Ayurvedic treatment. Each person is believed to have one or two dominant doshas, though the interplay of all three contributes to an individual's unique characteristics. This concept of classification based on individual

[85]Haasl-Blilie, Veena, 'Balancing Your Menstrual Cycle with Ayurveda: A Natural Approach,' *Saumya Ayurveda*, 22 August 2021, https://www.saumya-ayurveda.com/post/how-to-balance-your-menstrual-cycle-naturally-with-ayurveda.

doshas/body types helps in understanding human behaviour and emotions beyond gender differences. This helps in crafting personalized programmes for both the prevention and cure of ailments.

While many of the Sanskrit terms in Ayurveda might seem daunting at first, especially if we aren't familiar with the language, the pursuit of understanding and gaining mastery over our true self should be motivation enough to adopt this ancient system of medicine. The aim is to root ourselves ingratitude and find viable options to decode the secret of our bodies for healthy living by consciously incorporating food, work, rest, yoga and meditation into our daily routines that support and balance the doshas.

THE FUNCTIONS OF THE DOSHAS

All five elements play a crucial role in determining both emotional and physical health. It is essential to understand that each individual possesses a unique combination of vata, pitta and kapha.

Vata is characterized by the wind, and is related to bodily movements. This dosha is formed by the interaction of two elements—air/wind/vayu and space/akasa/ether. It is considered to be the most important dosha, overseeing functions such as the shedding of uterine blood, discharge of waste products and delivery of nutrients to the body's tissues.[86]

Pitta constitutes the transformative nature of fire (bile) energy and is related to temperament. This dosha is formed by the interaction of fire/agni and water /jal—the two contradictory elements vital for digestion and metabolism. It is

[86] Saini, Gurnam, 'Dysfunctional Uterine Bleeding Ayurveda Management', *Pure Herbal Ayurved Clinic*, https://www.pureherbalayurved.com.au/dysfuncational-uterine-bleeding-ayurveda-management.htm.

also responsible for maintaining body temperature and causes an increase in thirst and/or appetite when aggravated. It also plays a role in determining the onset, frequency and duration of menstruation.

Kapha embodies the cohesive nature of water (mucous), safeguards tissues and hydrates cells. This dosha is formed by the interaction of earth/prithvi and water/jal and acts as a lubricant for joints. It is also responsible for the body's immunity, sustenance, structuring and regular monthly cycle.

IDENTIFY YOUR DOSHAS

'Anyone who believes that anything can be
suited to everyone is a great fool,
because medicine is practised not on mankind in general,
but on every individual in particular.'

—HENRI DE MONDEVILLE

Globally, women can explore effective methods to maintain their health throughout their various phases of life, and the wisdom of Ayurveda offers valuable insights for mental and menstrual health enhancement.[87] If you are new to it, the first step would be to get your doshas assessed by a qualified *vaidya* or Ayurveda practitioner, as they can help in diagnosing individual doshas through pulse diagnosis (*nadi vigyan*), a technique for identifying the dosha by analysing physical, emotional, mental and behavioural imbalances.[88] This diagnosis reveals the root cause, forming the basis for tailor-made remedies.

[87] Dhimar, Deepika, Shailendra Kumar Janghel, and Prema Bhagat, 'A Review Study: Role of Ayurveda in Women's Life', *World Journal of Pharmaceutical and Medical Research*, Vol. 8, No. 6, 2022, 98–101.

[88] 'Nadi Pariksha or Pulse Diagnosis', *The Art of Living*, https://www.artofliving.org/in-en/ayurveda/remedies/nadi-pariksha-pulse-diagnosis.

Following are some of the characteristic traits that help identify doshas/body types:

Features	Vata	Pitta	Kapha
Body frame	Thin, tall, short, bony	Medium height, toned muscles, good metabolism	Large, broad, well-built, usually short and curvy
Weight	Low	Moderate	Heavy
Hair	Dry, dark, curly	Soft, oily, bald	Abundant, wavy, thick
Skin	Dry, rough, dull	Soft, oily, warm, acne, tan, freckles, moles, sensitive to heat	Thick, moist, cold, pale, fair
Eyes	Small, dull, dark, brown	Sharp, penetrating, poor vision	Large, expressive eyes
Hands	Cold, thin, dry	Medium, sweaty	Large, thick, round and oily
Appetite	Irregular, erratic, sparse, quick eater	Strong, regular habits, requires timely meals	Good, healthy appetite
Thirst	Varies at different times	Excessive	Minimal
Taste preferences	Sweet, sour, salty, oily, spicy	Sweet, bitter, raw, lightly spiced food	Pungent, bitter, food cooked with spices
Elimination	Scanty, dry, hard, constipated, gassy, painful	Soft, loose, burning sensation	Thick, slow, solid
Urination	Frequent, scanty, colourless	Yellow, warm, burning sensation	Average, milky, infrequent

Features	Vata	Pitta	Kapha
Sweat	Minimal, odourless, dislike cold climate, sensitive to cold wind and dry weather	Sweat profusely, pungent odour, dislike hot climate, sensitive to heat and humidity	Sensitive to cold and damp environments
Sleep	Light, restless, disturbed, suffers from insomnia	Sound and moderately good sleep	Heavy sleepers
Endurance	Low, poor endurance	Medium strength, can overexert	Strong, high endurance, low exertion
Finance	Earns and spends easily	Spends moderately and efficiently	Saves for rainy days
Season	Winter	Spring	Summer

To live our authentic selves, we need to understand our inherited and acquired behavioural patterns. Accepting ourselves and respecting others' patterns leads us to do similar tasks in diverse ways. Acknowledging each other's habits, tastes, preferences and endurance fosters compassion and harmony in our lives. The table below provides a broad overview of different physical, mental and emotional manifestations.

Features	Vata	Pitta	Kapha
Balanced mind	Inspired, energetic, adaptable, quick in action, highly spirited, good communicator, quick to grasp, enthusiastic, decision makers, creative, artistic and imaginative	Passionate, powerful, focused, intelligent, good leader, enlightened, courageous, warm, friendly, clever, motivated, easily succeeds	Loving, nurturing, stable, loyal, peaceful, forgiving, joyful, calm, content, easy-going, slow, deliberate, grounded, speaks and moves slowly
Imbalanced mind	Indecisive, agitated, secretive, anxious, talkative, unreliable, hyperactive, inconsistent, restless, rebellious, disorganized, lacks boundaries, unstable, rigid, unable to complete goals or take big decisions	Aggressive, reckless, proud, critical, angry, opinionated, snappy, holds grudges, over-ambitious	Insecure, materialistic, controlling, lonely, attached, lethargic, sad, slow, dull, clingy, inactive, avoids confrontation

Features	Vata	Pitta	Kapha
Imbalanced body	Dry skin, brittle hair and nails, anaemic, cramps, muscle spasms, constipation	Migraines, body aches, high blood pressure, indigestion, endometriosis	Obesity, pimples, allergy, sinus, congestion
Body parts	Dominates small and large intestine, colon; related to the nervous system	Dominates endocrine glands, liver, stomach, pancreas and eyes; related to digestion and metabolism	Dominates the chest, throat, lungs; related to strong immunity and body tissues
Memory	Learns and forgets quickly, short-term memory	Learns quickly and doesn't forget easily	Learns slowly and has a long-term memory

Ayurveda regards food as the most potent medicine and recommends dosha-appropriate diets as remedies to treat diseases affecting both mind and body. It is crucial to master the art of balancing emotions by choosing the right *guna* foods. Hence, what we consume directly affects our mental and emotional well-being. Scientific studies prove that eating nutrient-dense foods promotes the growth of beneficial gut bacteria.[89]

[89] Pelc, Corrie, 'Eating More Fruits and Vegetables Improves Gut Health, Study Shows,' *Medical News Today*, 2 November 2023, https://www.medicalnewstoday.com/articles/healthier-gut-microbiome-eat-more-fruit-vegetables#Fresh-fruits-and-vegetables-support-gut-health.

THE THREE GUNAS

Guna is a Sanskrit word that means 'quality/energy of food' and also describes a person's emotions, health, consciousness and behavioural traits. According to Sankhya philosophy, our dosha/prakriti manifests as gunas, which are further classified as three essential qualities: *sattvic* (vata), *rajasic* (pitta) and *tamasic* (kapha).

These three gunas are interconnected, constantly wavering and are present in everything (e.g., days and nights, seasons, situations and emotions). They are also present in individuals in varying proportions. Consumption of balanced foods and lifestyle changes embody the idea that these three gunas can make a person more stable, grounded and receptive to changes in life. Let us analyse the three gunas of food that are vital for daily consumption and play a specific and essential role in a woman's health and well-being.

Rajasic

Extremely flavoured, rich, creamy, bitter, sour, spicy and pungent food

These foods can stimulate passion, purpose, aggression and pain while promoting energy and positivity, which are essential for completing everyday tasks. They also build mental resilience. However, when consumed in excess, they may lead to overwhelming feelings of aggression, frustration and anger. Such foods are best consumed in moderate proportions as they are not easily digestible. Examples include whole pulses, dal, beans millet, buckwheat lentils; sour cream, yoghurt, fermented foods; nightshades like potato, eggplant, cayenne pepper and paprika; pickles, chillies and onions; refined sugar; and stimulants such as tea, coffee and aerated drinks. Note that heavily spiced, salted, overcooked food and even items prepared in anger can adopt a rajasic quality.

Tamasic

Highly processed, heavy, oily, cold and frozen food

Such foods diminish the body's energy, weaken its ability to fight diseases and disrupt the functioning of the immune system. They can lead to indigestion and hence become the epitome of inertia, making the body and mind dull, drowsy and lethargic. Additionally, they may cause depression, mood swings and unnatural cravings. When limited in consumption, tamasic food can be beneficial by preventing anxiety, aiding concentration and putting your mind at ease.

Examples include greasy fast foods, refined grains, canned and processed food and refined sugar. Alcohol, mushrooms, beef, sausages, ham, red meat, molasses and fermented, stale or leftover, reheated food, along with fruits that are overripe or not ripe enough also possess tamasic qualities. It is important to note that food prepared with indifference or overconsumption can also take on a tamasic nature.

Sattvic

Fresh, light, plant-based, nutrient-dense, naturally flavoured and alkaline food

These types of foods are a neutral force that purifies our minds and bodies and raises mental awareness. Hence, this is the guna that Ayurveda recommends as best suited for greater well-being. Sattvic food prepared with pure devotion brings lucidity to all thoughts and enables us to exercise the full potential of all functions.

Examples include yellow and green moong, yellow lentils, basmati rice, quinoa, vegetables (such as sweet potato, sprouts and leafy greens), sweet fruits (such as mango, dates and pears), ethically raised cow's milk, ghee, yoghurt, almonds, white sesame seeds, cashew, all herbs, spices (such as turmeric, fennel, cumin, coriander and saffron), natural sweeteners (such as jaggery, raw sugar and raw honey), and cold-pressed oils. One needs to note that all anti-inflammatory food, freshly-cooked food (which is consumed within 3–4 hours of its preparation) that is free of artificial colours and preservatives and food cooked with devotion and gratitude have sattvic properties.

Ayurveda recommends sattvic food due to its healing nature and ability to calm the mind and sharpen the intellect, and recommends complementing it with moderate consumption of rajasic and tamasic foods to incorporate vigour and stability.

The need to balance all three gunas in different ratios is essential as tamasic promotes the need for pause and restful sleep, rajasic adds zest to life and sattvic infuses peace and patience by raising human qualities.

While food choices can balance doshas to a great extent, Ayurveda emphasises synchronizing the body and mind with its circadian rhythm through scheduled nourishment and slumber cycles. A balanced inner clock aligned with daily routines ensures dosha equilibrium.

AN AYURVEDIC APPROACH

Women must introspect and take proactive measures to identify the root cause of menstrual imbalances, addressing them through a dosha-altering lifestyle along with dietary changes, to promote physical and emotional well-being.

Know Your Bleeding Pattern

Developing a positive attitude towards menstruation starts with the identification of bleeding patterns and menstrual abnormalities. Irregularities can then be correlated with the inherent traits of the respective doshas, as abnormalities occur only when doshas are imbalanced due to hormonal variations. For instance, an imbalance in vata may result in severe abdominal cramps, an imbalance in pitta could cause mood swings and an imbalance in kapha might result in heavy and clotted menstrual bleeding.

Doshas	Bleeding pattern	Discomfort	Emotions	Suggestions
Vata dosha imbalance	Scanty, irregular, delayed periods	Cramps in the lower abdomen	Anxiety, fear, poor appetite, mood swings	Take breaks to nourish and heal the body and mind
Pitta dosha imbalance	Medium flow, frequent clotting	Vomiting sensation, diarrhoea, acne, constipation, migraines	Anger, irritability	Relax and pause in between work to nurture and express creatively
Kapha dosha imbalance	Heavy flow, dark, thick, red clots	Water retention, bloating, yeast infections	Depression, binge eating	Avoid oversleeping and let go of negative emotions

Menstruation requires self-care and should not be viewed as an illness. The *Sushruta Samhita* (the ancient Sanskrit text on medicine and surgery) states that abnormal menstruation is caused by disturbed vata, pitta and kapha and can be reversed by establishing a healthy lifestyle and adopting holistic methods tailored to the age and nature of an individual.

Healing Herbs and Spices

'Every time you eat or drink,
you are either feeding disease or fighting it.'

—HEATHER MORGAN

Herbs are among the most effective ways to balance hormonal variations. The use of medicinal herbs and plants in food and for treating ailments represents one of the oldest and purest forms of healing. What could be better than treating imbalances of particular doshas with concoctions prepared from the ingredients already present in our kitchens? Herbs and spices hold a cherished place in every household, especially in India, where age-old ancestral recipes are still used as home remedies for all kinds of health issues.

These small wonders are powerhouses of energy that can boost immunity, increase metabolism, aid weight loss, address skin problems, regularize menstrual flow and ease menstrual cramps. Ayurveda recommends the inclusion of herbs and spices regularly in all forms of cooking as they have little or no side effects. Their benefits can be maximized when consumed in the right combinations and proportions, for which one needs to approach professional practitioners.

A few magical ingredients and their benefits to balance your dosha:

- Fennel (*saunf*) is known to alleviate menstrual cramps and minimize bloating.
- Fenugreek (*methi*) offers relief from menstrual pain.

- Cumin (*jeera*) helps regulate body temperature and boost gut health.
- Cinnamon (*dalchini*) supports weight loss and regulates menstrual flow.
- Black pepper (*kaali mirch*) stimulates digestive secretions and aids in toxin elimination.
- Basil (*tulsi*) leaves are a potent antioxidant.
- Mint (*pudina*) leaves provide relaxation for muscle cramps.
- Rose (*gulab*) petals improve blood circulation and relieve discomfort.
- Ginger (*adrak*) and turmeric (*haldi*) have anti-inflammatory properties.

Teas and Infusions

Authentic herb and spice concoctions are packed with unique antioxidants, making them highly effective in aiding digestion. Regular consumption can also help balance menstrual cycles. These concoctions are simple preparations and can easily be incorporated into daily routines, and consumed in between meals, after meals or throughout the day. Women who are pregnant or lactating must seek the advice of a medical professional before consuming these concoctions.

Vata Tea (a concoction to balance vata during menstruation)

Fennel (*saunf*) seeds	1 tsp
Carom (*ajwain*) seeds	¼ tsp
Coriander (*dhania*) seeds	1 tsp
Fenugreek (*methi*) seeds	½ tsp
Ginger (*adrak*) ground or grated	¼ tsp
Clove (*laung*)	1 piece
Mint (*pudina*)	2–4 leaves
Lime (*nimbu*)	Half a piece

Jaggery (*gud*) or natural sweetener	To taste (optional)

Kapha Tea (a concoction to be had during the follicular phase)

Cinnamon (*dalchini*)/ground	1 stick/1 tsp
Ginger (*adrak*) powder	¼ tsp
Fresh Ginger (*adrak*) crushed	¼ tsp
Clove (*laung*)	1 piece
Turmeric (*haldi*) powder	¼ tsp
Dried basil (*tulsi*) leaves	1 tsp
Black pepper (*kaali mirch*)	¼ tsp
Honey (*shahad*)	To taste (optional)

Pitta Tea (a concoction to balance Pitta during the ovulatory and luteal phases)

Cumin (*jeera*) seeds	½ tsp
Fennel (*saunf*) seeds	1 tsp
Turmeric (*haldi*) powder	¼ tsp
Ginger (*adrak*) powder	A pinch
Cardamom (*elaichi*)	A pinch
Saffron (*kesar*)	2 or 3 strands
Coriander (*dhania*) and mint (*pudina*) leaves	A few
Rose (*gulab*) petals (dried)	A few
Jaggery (*gud*)	To taste (optional)

METHOD

The process of making traditional, herbal concoctions usually involves boiling 200 ml of water and adding crushed seeds, spices and any additional ingredients. Once the mixture has simmered for 5–10 minutes, fresh herbs are added and allowed to infuse for a few minutes before consumption. To enhance the flavour, consider adding lime, honey or jaggery. Taking turmeric and pepper together can also increase the absorption of nutrients. For a more convenient approach, grind all dry ingredients into a coarse powder that can easily be added to hot water for daily consumption.

In different parts of the world, various herbs such as motherwort, yarrow, wild yam, chasteberry, chamomile and Chinese herbs like dong quai and bai shao are commonly used to treat menstrual problems. These traditional healing practices passed down from our ancestors are valuable resources that should be preserved, practised and promoted to safeguard the well-being of future generations.

THE BOTTOM LINE

Do not let genetics hinder you from leading a healthy lifestyle. It is the choices you make at every moment that significantly impact your life. While ignorance and a reckless attitude can lead to sickness and a troubled mind, wisdom and a mindful attitude result in a sound mind and a healthy body.

The younger generation should recognize the futility of conforming to a superficial image or lifestyle. Instead of attempting to alter your body, shift your perspective by treating your body with care and compassion, aiming for better menstrual and mental health. This approach will help you become a better version of yourself.

NIMMI'S MANTRA

Treat your body with kindness and respect, as it is the only one you have in this lifetime.

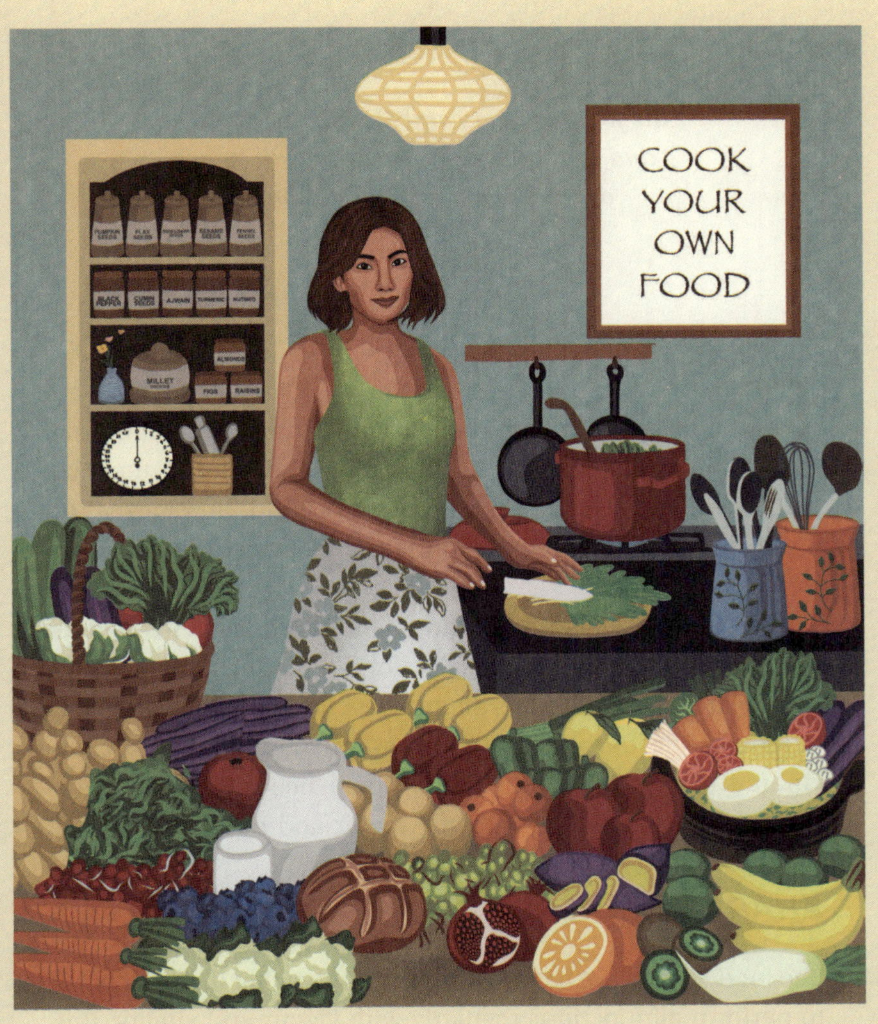
COOK
YOUR
OWN
FOOD
BLACK PEPPER
CUMIN SEEDS
AJWAIN
TURMERIC
MILLET
RAISINS

10
THE FOOD FACTOR

'The food you eat can be either the safest and most powerful form of medicine or the slowest form of poison.'

—ANN WIGMORE

Food is omnipresent in our day-to-day life, defining an individual's culture, beliefs and heritage all around the world. Our forefathers respected food—the sustenance of life—with an attitude of gratitude towards Mother Earth. But have you ever wondered about the significance of food for our well-being?

Since the dawn of civilization, food has been venerated as a cornerstone of human health, forging connections among people in all cultural celebrations. Despite its regional diversity in terms of flavour, colour and tradition, food has always been curated to meet the body's nutritional needs, providing the essential fuel for energy, growth, repair and metabolism.

AHARA AS ENERGY

The food (ahara) we eat provides the energy that fuels the body to perform all functions regularly with vigour and vitality. It is necessary to include food with different types of energy or life (*prana*) for each cycle to support hormonal variations. These variations can stem from circumstances, individuals, climate fluctuations, traumas, illnesses and other factors.

It is important to be mindful of the impact that different foods and pairings of food can have on our bodies and health. Not all foods are equally beneficial for everyone because of differences in digestion and body type, which can influence how food is processed and metabolized in the body. Some food pairings can have a soothing effect, aiding in digestion and promoting balance between the body and mind, while other pairings may cause allergies or intolerances, leading to discomfort and disease.

Emphasizing the effects of food on our health in every individual, Ayurvedic principles stress the importance of customizing the diet as per our unique body type or dosha to achieve optimal well-being. Instead of viewing food as simply good or bad, recognize it as energy that can either nourish or hinder our health. By transforming our perception towards food and making informed decisions, we can uplift our overall health and standard of living.

It is important to acknowledge that our emotional and mental well-being plays a significant role in our digestive health. An anxious or depressed mind can lead to poor dietary choices that, in turn, can result in digestive issues and contribute to the development of metabolic disorders. Therefore, working on our emotional health is an essential step in maintaining healthy eating habits and reversing these conditions. By developing willpower, commitment, discipline and common sense with respect to our diets, we can promote a healthier and more balanced approach to food and improve our digestive health.

THE PSYCHOLOGY OF *RASA*

'Let food be your first medicine
and the kitchen your first pharmacy.'

—TAITTIRIYA UPANISHAD

In today's world, there is a rising trend of eating mindlessly. This lack of mind and body connection is often referred to as eating amnesia due to acquired food habits over time. Sadly, it leads to poor nutritional choices and weight gain.

Being mindful of our emotions is crucial when considering our food choices, as they often stem from unresolved issues that impact our physical well-being. By tracking our daily food intake, we can cultivate greater control over our thoughts, rectify unhealthy dietary choices, and shift towards nourishing food and wholesome habits to revitalize our lives.

The Ayurvedic concept of food includes six basic tastes (*rasas*)—sweet, salty, sour, pungent, astringent and bitter,[90] which has a distinct and direct effect on the psychological disposition of individuals. It also asserts that consuming all six tastes daily in varied proportions is essential for feeling satiated and energetic.

Thus, through mindful eating, along with necessary lifestyle changes, sufficient rest and appropriate yogic practices, you too can give your body self-healing properties. Each taste has a specific purpose and consuming them in the right proportions can optimize internal mechanisms to heal ailments naturally. If including all flavours in every meal is not feasible, incorporating them into at least one meal daily, preferably lunch, can be beneficial to the body. This inclusion is also vital for the

[90]Eisler, Melissa, 'The 6 Tastes of Ayurveda', *Chopra*, 16 May 2016, https://chopra.com/blogs/ayurveda/the-6-tastes-of-ayurveda.

healthy functioning of the reproductive organs, as taste is associated with Svadhisthana (Womb) Chakra—the powerful centre for pleasure, gratification and preservation (as detailed in Chapter 14).

A deficiency in any of these six tastes can lead to over-indulgence, which can disrupt the secretion of hormones. Understanding the science behind these tastes reveals that the right combination of different foods ultimately provides sustenance.[91]

FOODS FOR YOUR HORMONES

The delicate interplay between food and hormones is crucial in maintaining a harmonious physiological balance. Fluctuations in reproductive hormones can have a profound impact on our emotions, underscoring the importance of the tailored nutritional requirements necessary for hormonal stability. Recognizing the symptoms of hormonal imbalance allows for a nuanced understanding of the four distinct phases of the menstrual cycle, guiding the inclusion of supportive food patterns.

Phase 1: Menstrual Phase/Inner Winter (Days 1-5)

Dosha: Vata (Wind Element)

Hormones: Oestrogen is at its lowest, so it is natural to feel low during this phase.

Symptoms: Headache, skin dryness, severe fatigue, sweet cravings, acne breakout and cramps.

Care: During this menstrual phase, *apana vayu* (the downward-

[91]Mukta, Shiva Kumar Harti, and Mangalagowri V. Rao, 'Role of Rasas and their Order of Intake in Nutrition,' Vol. 6, No. 2, 2019, 266–269. https://storage.googleapis.com/journal-uploads/ejpmr/article_issue/1548934205.pdf.

moving wind energy governing menstrual bleeding) is in motion. The uterus actively sheds its lining, which has to be supported with nourishing food and rest. Vata (wind) is highly active and sends out certain signals to slow down. If these warnings are disregarded over time, they can manifest as PMS, insomnia, constipation or digestive problems in the subsequent cycles.

Healing foods: Nourish yourself with nutrient-dense, iron-rich and sattvic food during this phase; for example, 'Havishya anna' (rice) meal made from rice, ghee and milk. Cleanse, soak, and wash the rice thoroughly before boiling it with milk. Enhance the flavour with jaggery or sugar and cardamom powder.

- Inner winter calls for high-quality, vegetarian protein sources, healthy fats, organic dairy (milk, ghee and butter from the native cow); opt for A2 milk (for easy digestion), organic eggs, wild-caught oily fish, nut butter and avocado.
- Warm, sattvic food, such as moong dal khichdi, rice puddings, nourishing beverages and thick vegetable soups are light on the stomach and easy to digest.
- Khichdi: Our good old khichdi from the Indian kitchen has become extremely popular all over the world for its restorative and nourishing properties. It can be easily prepared by cooking half a cup of washed and soaked basmati rice or millet and half a cup of yellow lentils (yellow moong dal) together in four cups of water. A variety of washed and cut organic vegetables or vegetable broth can be added for nutrition, along with spices like turmeric, cumin, fresh ginger, pepper, saunf, curry leaves and asafoetida. Flavour with native cow ghee or sesame oil for added richness and curative properties.
- Keep your body replenished and energetic with iron-rich foods, such as lentils, pumpkin seeds, spinach, lean protein, millets, dry prunes, berries, beets, watermelon, cucumber and kale.

- Indian herbs and seasonings can help in proper assimilation, while indulging in homemade sweets made with jaggery or natural sugars or chocolates with 70% cacao content can help curb unhealthy sugar cravings.
- Probiotics like ginger, lemon or chamomile and honey can ease cramps, heavy flow, exhaustion and body pain, improving gut health.
- Algae and omega supplements provide additional health benefits.

Cravings and low moods depict imbalances in bio-energies. It would be wise to avoid packaged, processed meat or heavy, oily, salty, cold and sugar-rich foods. Reduce or eliminate alcohol, caffeine and smoking during menstruation.

Phase 2: Follicular Phase/Inner Spring (Days 6–11)

Dosha: Kapha (Water Element)

Hormones: This is the inner-spring period when oestrogen and progesterone are on the rise. The FSHs slightly increase their secretions around this time by preparing and strengthening the body for probable conception.

Symptoms: General heaviness may be experienced.

Care: There is a heightened need for energizing nutrients during this phase, necessitating proper support for the body.

Healing food: Energy-boosting food.

- Nourish the body with anti-inflammatory and protein-rich food, including free-range chicken, salmon, organic eggs, sprouts, non-dairy and plant-based protein such as oats, nuts, cashews and flax seeds, to increase oestrogen production.
- Savour sautéed, steamed or stir-fried organic food, cooked with colourful vegetables like carrots, spinach, sprouts and

avocado. Enjoy with raw sauerkraut or pickled veggies for added sustenance.

- Incorporate Indian spices, such as cinnamon, pepper, ginger, cardamom and turmeric, into warm concoctions during this period.
- Increasing the intake of quality fats from fish, coconut oil, avocado and flax seeds can strengthen immunity.
- Consider supplements like shatavari to stimulate oestrogen production.

Other lifestyle changes such as waking up early, avoiding daytime napping and staying active throughout the day can help keep the kapha dosha in balance. Indulge in relaxation with salt scrubs or sesame oil massages.

Phase 3: Ovulatory Phase/Inner Summer (Days 12–19)

Dosha: Pitta (Fire Element)

Hormones: Oestrogen is at its highest, with energy, sex drive and motivation peaking during this inner summer phase.

Symptoms: Acne, oily skin, body odour, heaviness and high libido.

Care: Pitta or fire dosha plays a significant role in the third and fourth (ovulatory and luteal) phases of the menstrual cycle. Pitta levels naturally rise to facilitate the ovulation process, leading to a rise in body temperature too.

Healing foods: Balancing carbs and proteins.

- A surge in oestrogen provides an energy boost while simultaneously curbing hunger. This reduced appetite may lead to increased cravings for carbohydrates, as they serve as a quick source of energy.
- Choosing protein-rich food with fibre can help balance

the pitta and support liver function. Increasing the intake of lentils and peas, leafy greens and vegetables, including okra, spinach, cabbage and broccoli, can induce bile juices and help with digestion.

- Fresh fruits such as papaya and pineapple, refreshing salads, peppermint tea, coconut water and lemon water can help with liver cleansing.
- It is wise to feed gut bacteria by adding more high-fibre and fermented foods to your diet. Consuming yoghurt, miso, kefir, kimchi or kombucha, along with sauerkraut or fermented vegetables as well as prebiotics such as veggies, legumes, peas, berries and asparagus can boost gut health and aid in liver detoxification.
- Consider incorporating follicular-friendly superfoods like spirulina, milk thistle supplements, sesame or sunflower seeds, aloe vera and turmeric into your diet.

For people concerned about weight issues, this phase presents an opportunity for natural detoxification by incorporating liver-friendly foods, intense training and mindful fasting.

Phase 4: Luteal Phase/Inner Monsoon/Fall (Days 20–26)

Dosha: Pitta (Fire Element)

Hormones: This is the inner monsoon/fall phase when progesterone peaks and subsequently drops towards the end of the cycle, bringing down energy levels and resulting in mood swings, depression and PMS.

Symptoms: Tenderness in breasts, temporary water retention and bloating, insomnia, acne and experiencing emotions such as anxiety, anger and irritability.

Care: External factors such as stress, over-expectations, over-enthusiasm and overwork can influence hormones intensely during this phase. The most effective remedy for repairing and rebuilding the body is high-quality sleep, coupled with self-kindness by releasing ungrateful thoughts.

Healing foods: Opt for light and nutrient-rich, small, frequent meals that are rich in magnesium.

- Rice and vegetables seasoned with spices, healthy vegetable cutlets or rolls can soothe one's palate and manage bloating. Starchy vegetables such as pumpkin and sweet potatoes are also good options.
- Cereals such as bajra, jowar, barley, rice and steel-cut oats; figs, dates and walnuts; sunflower seeds, spices and herbs such as ginger, mint, turmeric, garlic, long pepper and bay leaf; sugar-based products such as jaggery, honey and A2 dairy products can ease PMS symptoms.
- Consume magnesium-rich foods such as bananas, almonds, dark chocolates, quinoa, avocados, leafy vegetables, yoghurt and kefir to increase serotonin levels, thereby preventing migraine attacks.
- Enjoy water-rich fruits such as strawberries, watermelon, grapes, melons and cucumber, lime juice, tender coconut, millets, apples and crunchy sesame/peanut bars to promote smooth bowel movements. Fruits like guavas are also great alternatives.
- Consider drinking apple cider vinegar mixed with warm water before bed to improve gut health, regulate blood sugar levels, release bile and aid digestion.
- Ayurvedic supplements like ashwagandha, aloe vera and Brahmi are highly recommended.
- Consider drinking a comforting glass of warm turmeric milk, a cherished Indian tradition often enjoyed at night. This soothing elixir can be particularly beneficial in calming the

nerves during this phase. Milk (derived from grass-fed native cows) mixed with haldi has been a traditional remedy for centuries in Indian households. It is now widely recognized for its numerous health benefits and is commonly consumed before bedtime, particularly combined with black pepper for the enhanced bioavailability of curcumin. The addition of jaggery, ginger and saffron not only provides a delicious taste but also promotes relaxation and restful sleep. This warm and nutritious beverage possesses powerful antioxidants and antibacterial and anti-fungal properties that can boost immunity, improve digestion and enhance gut health. According to Ayurveda, it is considered a sattvic drink with medicinal value, balancing the three doshas.

Research indicates that the milk from ethically raised grass-fed cows contains unique micronutrients that offer superior taste and health benefits as compared to plant-based or hormone-injected dairy milk.[92]

Women should be mindful of low progesterone levels, which may cast shadows upon the levels of serotonin. Decreased levels of happy hormones can give rise to PMS symptoms and negative emotions such as mood swings, anger and depression. It can also increase cravings for high-calorie, processed food; sugar treats; and stimulants such as coffee, alcohol, spicy food, sodas and colas; all seem appealing but can easily upset the digestion process, impacting menstrual and mental health.

The urge to eat convenient, fast foods can be set right by disciplining the mind and consuming natural and homemade foods that are rich in Vitamin B, magnesium and calcium.

[92]Devje, Shahzadi, 'Grass-fed Milk: Everything You Need to Know', *Healthline*, Healthline Media, 24 January 2022, https://www.healthline.com/nutrition/grass-fed-milk.

Adding supplements to the diet can balance the levels of progesterone hormone.

Thus, preparing for a positive, painless period begins in the luteal phase and relies on the preceding ovulation phase. This cycle of interdependency embodies the graceful rhythm of nurturing well-being.

Embracing a diet rich in healthy fats, lean proteins, essential fatty acids, fibre, minerals and complex carbohydrates ensures access to vital nutrients. A balanced meal is a snapshot of a diet that covers the three core food groups—a quarter of carbohydrates, a quarter of proteins and half of vegetables.

THE ELIMINATION PROCESS

One of the most common complaints of women just before their periods is constipation; proper elimination is essential for the body to function optimally. Fluctuations in progesterone and oestrogen, along with certain health conditions or medications, may contribute to this symptom. However, constipation is a typical occurrence just before the onset of periods. Adding prebiotics or insoluble fibres to the diet can ease the discomfort by preventing overgrowth of bad bacteria and promoting good gut health as a proper diet inclusive of cabbage, snake gourd, carrot, potato, radish, onion, ash gourd, drumstick, banana (medium ripe), oats, berries, leek, asparagus, leafy greens and soaked chia seeds can facilitate bowel movements.

Drinking buttermilk or warm water after meals or consuming herbal concoctions throughout the day can aid in digestion. Chewing betel (or *paan*) leaves or betel nut with slaked lime and clove after meals is an age-old Indian custom known for its curative and digestive properties, still practised in many households today. Lifestyle modifications, combined with the practice of *Pawanmuktasana* (a yoga pose aimed at relieving digestive discomfort) and regular brisk walks, can provide relief. However, if the issue persists, it is advisable to seek professional assistance for serious medical conditions such as rectal prolapse; further, a proper diagnosis and consultation with nutritional specialists can guide you in the right direction.

THE INCONVENIENCE OF CONVENIENT FOODS

We are witnessing an increase in the mass production of 'convenient foods' containing synthetic, preservative ingredients that can be highly toxic. Frozen and processed, ready-to-eat 'fast foods' are enticing the current generation to work more, do more and be more at the cost of depriving the human body of nutritious food and much-needed rest and sleep.[93,94]

Increasingly, busy individuals are relying on convenient foods produced in factories rather than foods made with wholesome, real ingredients. The substitution of natural and real ingredients with ready-to-eat alternatives is eroding cooking skills, dulling taste buds with artificial flavours and creating a culture of sick people who believe in 'sick care' than proactive healthcare, regardless of the prevalence of diet books and trendy dietary plans. This shift has become more

[93]Huzar, Timothy, 'Is Fast Food Bad for You? All You Need to Know About Its Nutrition and Impacts,' *Medical News Today*, Healthline Media, 9 February 2023, https://www.medicalnewstoday.com/articles/324847.

[94]Rahkovsky, Ilya, Young Jo, and Andrea Carlson, 'What Drives Consumers to Purchase Convenience Foods?,' *US Department of Agriculture*, 24 July 2018, https://www.usda.gov/media/blog/2018/07/24/what-drives-consumers-purchase-convenience-foods.

common due to hectic lifestyles and time constraints, leading to serious nutritional deficiencies, adversely affecting health and longevity.

The consumption of unhealthy food can lead to inflammation, while accumulated undigested metabolic waste can gradually weaken the digestive system, leading to hormonal imbalances, reproductive health complications, Type 2 diabetes, cancer and heart diseases. Many chronic ailments stem from prolonged exposure to poor dietary choices, toxic ingredients, heavily processed food, nutritional deficiencies and unhealthy lifestyle habits developed over a long period of time.

It is essential that modern eating habits are modified based on an individual's age, nature of work and weather conditions. These subtle adjustments can make a great difference, yielding significant benefits. Moreover, a woman needs to be aware of the different phases of menstruation, pregnancy, motherhood and other health concerns to tailor her diet effectively.

GUT HEALTH MATTERS

As mentioned previously, every cycle is interdependent and influences the following cycle. Food does affect our hormones. So the mantra here is to feed your gut bacteria with fibre-rich and healthy unsaturated fats that combat inflammation, thereby significantly reducing menstrual pain.

Research indicates that 90% of diseases arise from the gut due to poor eating habits and incompatible food combinations.[95] Further, women may experience reproductive hormonal disorders due to demanding work pressures, diverse

[95]Liang, Linda, Clarissa Saunders, and Nerses Sanossian, 'Food, Gut Barrier Dysfunction, and Related Diseases: A New Target for Future Individualized Disease Prevention and Management', *Food Science & Nutrition*, Vol. 11, No. 4, 2023, 1671–1704, https://doi.org/10.1002%2Ffsn3.3229.

addictions, inadequate sleep, stress, mental health issues, high expectations, improper breathing and unhealthy food choices, including eating disorders.

Be mindful, as all these factors can impact reproductive hormones. Variations in oestrogen levels influence gut health significantly by bringing down immunity levels. Hence, women must take care of their gut health. Studies show that a significant portion of the body's serotonin supply is produced by gut bacteria, and gets suppressed due to chronic stress, causing digestive issues.[96]

Choosing nutritional diet plans and personalizing them based on the body's doshas can contribute to overall health. A healthy gut heals its damaged lining by boosting energy levels. Once gut health improves, you are on the path to experiencing a healthy menstrual cycle.

NOURISH YOUR GUT BACTERIA

'Good gut health begets good overall health'

—DR TRACEY MARKS

Dr Tracey Marks, renowned psychiatrist, emphasizes the significance of our gut, stating, 'Our gut houses a lot of genetic material in its cells, influencing many of our body's functions in definite ways.' She recommends that we include high-fibre and fermented food in our diet to stimulate the gut microbiome population (also referred to as the second brain or secondary immune system).[97]

---

[96] Carpenter, Siri, 'That Gut Feeling', *Monitor on Psychology*, Vol. 43, No. 8, 2012, 50, https://www.apa.org/monitor/2012/09/gut-feeling.

[97] How Your Gut Bacteria Controls Your Mood, YouTube, https://www.youtube.com/watch?v=5h3Y4iNcN8g.

By incorporating natural, gut-friendly, pre and probiotics, you are aiding easy absorption of vital enzymes, thus ensuring that minimal or no toxins are produced and the body can use proteins efficiently. Probiotics are live microorganisms found in fermented foods. They promote a conducive environment for gut bacteria to thrive and offer numerous health benefits. For instance, an Indian fermented rice drink called *kanji* can be prepared by soaking half a cup of cooked rice overnight in two cups of water in a clay pot and consumed the next morning. You can add chopped onion, coriander and pink salt to enhance the flavour.

Both pre and probiotics can be consumed in their natural form or through supplements. So take care of your microbiome population by stocking up on fermented foods like yoghurt, pickles, peanut curd, sourdough bread, miso, kefir, kimchi or kombucha, along with pasteurized sauerkraut or fermented vegetables. Other prebiotic foods such as veggies, legumes, peas, berries, walnuts, oats, bananas, seafood and asparagus can further promote the growth of beneficial bacteria.

THE DYNAMICS OF EATING

'Thou should eat to live; not live to eat.'

—SOCRATES

It is essential to recognize the difference between 'need' and 'want' with respect to food. Health is dependent more on habits and structured lifestyles than on medicine. Hence, mastering healthy food habits can impact positively, reflecting on our emotional aspects too.

Mindful Planning

Plan for 2–3 wholesome meals a day based on the nature of your work and body requirements. A menu rich in nutrition, fibre and micronutrients makes it easily digestible and sustainable. Noon is the optimal time to incorporate all six flavours into your diet as our digestion ('digestive fire') mimics the sun's cycle. Biologically, noon is the time when blood sugar levels are regulated. The gut microbiome or the digestive fire is the strongest during this time, and hence it is best to keep lunch as the main meal of the day.

Adhering to a consistent meal schedule promotes optimal digestion and imbues one with boundless energy and vitality. Ignoring the body's cravings for nourishment and sustenance can result in fatigue, bodily aches and digestive issues. Healthy eating is a dynamic and transformative journey, shaped by a multitude of personal and cultural factors, including menstrual cycles, metabolic needs, habits, traditions and determination.

Mindful Cooking

Many traditions still regard cooking and eating as sacred ceremonial acts. By preparing your meals, you take charge of your health every day. This ensures control over the ingredients used, the calorie consumption and the freshness quotient, ensuring that the health of your entire family is taken care of. Further, mindful cooking also prevents wastage by preparing the right quantity and avoiding consuming nutrient-depleted leftovers.

The method of preparing food greatly influences its taste and the preservation of its nutrients. Slow cooking enhances flavour while using the right ingredients and cooking in earthenware or cast-iron utensils prevents harmful chemicals from being introduced into the food. Food absorbs energy, and negative emotions while cooking can negatively impact digestion as the energy or life force (prana) can transfer from the cook to food.[98] This energy can also be destroyed by overcooking, charring or deep-frying.

As a first step towards a healthier lifestyle, cultivate the habit of cooking food with real ingredients. Choose a variety of colourful fruits and vegetables, and cook simple dishes with fewer ingredients. You can follow your mother's recipes or explore recipe books. It is important to preserve traditional food habits and cook food in traditional, food-grade vessels infused with positive thoughts, which can heal and rejuvenate you.

Mindful Eating

The mastery of correct eating practices is fundamental for optimal digestion. The digestive system is regulated by the autonomic nervous system, meaning our thoughts have a direct impact on our digestion.[99] Therefore, it is crucial to recognize that the gut is constantly susceptible to both positive and negative emotions.

Before each meal, take a few deep breaths to cultivate tranquillity. Chew your food slowly, relishing each bite mindfully, paying attention to the colour, texture, aroma, flavour and taste. Eating requires a resolute and disciplined mindset, focused on fully embracing the experience with all senses.

Your posture and the right frame of mind are also powerful aids that help you relish food without stress. Sitting cross-

[98] 'Do Positive or Negative Thoughts while Cooking Get Transferred to the Food?', *The Times of India*, Bennett, Coleman & Co. Ltd., 21 April 2020, https://timesofindia.indiatimes.com/life-style/health-fitness/diet/do-positive-or-negative-thoughts-while-cooking-get-transferred-to-the-food/articleshow/75254336.cms.

[99] Cherpak, Christine E., 'Mindful Eating: A Review of How the Stress-Digestion-Mindfulness Triad May Modulate and Improve Gastrointestinal and Digestive Function', *Integrative Medicine*, Vol. 18, No. 4, 2019, 48–53, PMID: 32549835; PMCID: PMC7219460.

legged enhances the energies of the abdomen by increasing blood circulation. Be mindful to avoid topics related to illness, trauma, emotionally charged discussions or problems of the self or others during meals, as they all have the power to adversely affect the digestion process.

Consuming anything cold during meals can dampen the gut health (fire) and cause indigestion. Instead, drink warm, herbal concoctions between and after meals. They help digestive enzymes in absorbing foods and curb unhealthy cravings between meals.

Avoid multitasking during meals, such as engaging in activities like reading, watching television, working or using gadgets as you absorb unwanted energy from the digital media.[100] Mindful eating involves paying attention to portion control, establishing a regular meal schedule and being fully present during each meal. Keeping a food journal is an effective way to stay aware of your food habits and understand your eating behaviours.

Maintain low insulin levels by allowing adequate time between meals. Refrain from eating out of boredom; engage in gentle physical activity after meals. Eating when hungry and drinking when thirsty promotes healing. Understanding the dynamics of food makes it a powerful form of medicine.

Centenarians believe that achieving both wisdom and robust health requires a mindful approach to festive feasting. They advocate avoiding processed foods, sweets, pastries made from white refined flour as well as high-carbohydrate, high-fat and animal-based ingredients—often referred to as comfort foods. If consuming such foods cannot be avoided, they should

[100] Das, Rupam, 'Why Watching TV, and Mobile while Eating Is Becoming Surging Life Killer?,' *Lyfas Life Care*, Royal News Magazine, 25 November 2022, https://lyfas.com/uncategorized/why-watching-mobile-while-eating-is-becoming-surging-life-killer/rupam_lyfas/.

be done so in moderation, followed by warm water, green tea or yoghurt with roasted cumin to aid digestion. To prevent bloating, gas and indigestion, it is advisable to incorporate fibre-rich foods into the next meal of the day to counterbalance the effects of processed foods.

Compatible Food Combinations

It is crucial to recognize that the significance of food consumption lies not only in what is eaten but also in understanding the correlation and proportion of intake. Ayurveda, grounded in the vital energy (prana) of each food item, offers universally relevant principles, techniques and customs. However, it is imperative to acknowledge that they stand in stark contrast to contemporary dietary theories.

As per the principles of Ayurveda, conventional food pairings can significantly increase nutrition manifold and dramatically improve digestion.[101] Optimal combinations sustain energy and keep you active for a long time.

Some compatible food combinations include:

- Beans with grains, nuts, seeds and vegetables.
- Butter, ghee and cheese with grains, vegetables, beans, fish and cooked fruits.
- Leafy greens with tomatoes.
- Fruits of the same family, such as citrus, apples or melons.
- Milk is best enjoyed alone but can be combined with oatmeal and rice pudding or in the form of date milkshakes.

[101]'Ayurvedic Food Combining,' *Banyan Botanicals*, https://www.banyanbotanicals.com/info/ayurvedic-living/living-ayurveda/diet/ayurvedic-food-combining/.

Incompatible Food Combinations

Food can act as either an antidote or poison depending on its combinations.[102] Incompatible food pairings can lead to toxic build-ups resulting in multiple health complications. The gut, which transforms food into energy, gets disturbed when two foods that have opposing qualities are consumed together. Additionally, certain foods provide optimal nutrition only when eaten at specific times of the day. For example, yoghurt or curd may be excellent natural probiotics but consuming them at night can trigger mucous build-ups and chest congestion. While fruits eaten in the morning or a few hours before lunch offer a wealth of nutrition, pairing them with pulses or cereals can lead to acidity and heartburn. This is because fresh fruits can be digested quickly and combining them with slow-digesting cooked food leads to fermentation, bloating and disruptions in the gut microbiome.

According to the principles of Ayurveda, certain food combinations should be avoided to maintain optimal gut health and prevent diseases.

- Fruits with milk such as milkshakes.
- Fruits from the melon family should be eaten alone without combining them with other fruits.
- Mixing proteins with fats.
- Tea or coffee with savouries.
- Milk with yoghurt, cheese, sour fruits, fish, eggs, meat, beans, radish or nightshade veggies.
- Yoghurt or curds with tomatoes and cucumber.
- Mixing different types of proteins.

[102] Ayush, 'Ayurveda Shares Wrong Food Combinations! Are You Consuming Those?', *Ministry of Ayush*, Government of India, https://ayushnext.ayush.gov.in/detail/post/ayurveda-shares-wrong-food-combinations-are-you-consuming-those.

- Fruits and vegetables must be consumed separately for better digestion.

Ayurveda philosophy does not categorize food as inherently good or bad. It emphasizes that each food is digested at a different pace. Hence, combining fast and slow-digesting food can burden the digestive tract and should be mindfully avoided. Ayurveda stresses the various properties of food and suggests avoiding certain combinations for optimal wellness.

Indigestion is a prevalent ailment that plagues a majority of individuals at some point in their lives. This condition has the potential to drastically alter one's overall state of mind due to its detrimental effects on the body's functionality. Dr Swami Shankardevananda's insightful book, *The Practices of Yoga for the Digestive System*[103] provides a wealth of knowledge on digestive wellness, promoting awareness and fostering positive habits for a greater physical and emotional equilibrium.

THE BOTTOM LINE

In modern times, especially in urban areas, the quality of food is never fully in our control. However, we can control the quantity and intake, as healthcare is ultimately our responsibility. It requires exercising willpower and discipline to voluntarily educate ourselves and promote a healthy relationship with food.

Practising meditation increases the power of the Manipura or Solar Plexus Chakra, located two inches above the navel—the subtle life force connected with fire energy, which can influence metabolism and improve digestion. Consuming nutritious food, getting adequate rest, exercising and following the circadian rhythms can help eliminate toxins and free radicals, thereby

[103]Shankardevananda, Swami, *The Practices of Yoga for the Digestive System*, Yoga Publications Trust, Rishikesh, 1 January 2006.

improving digestion and immunity levels, which, in turn, enhance reproductive health.

NIMMI'S MANTRA

Make informed choices for a healthy relationship with food.

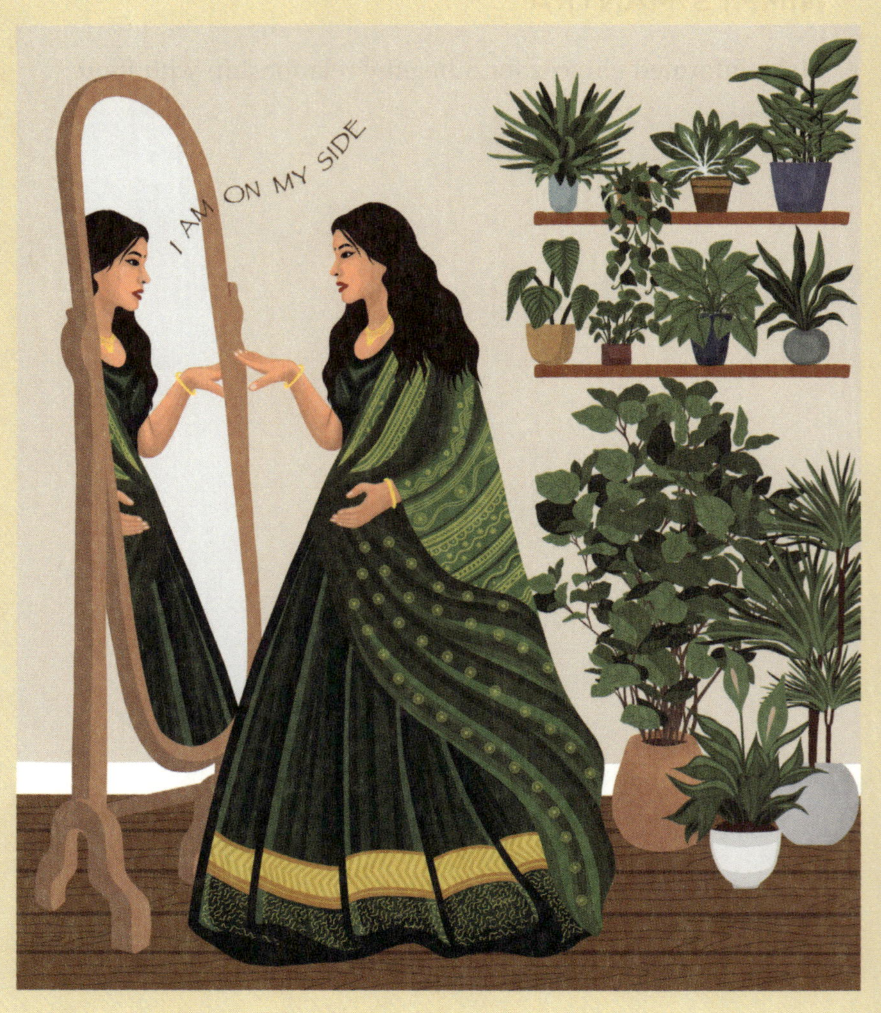
I AM ON MY SIDE

11

SUPPLEMENTING THE CREATIVE FORCE

'Your lack of confidence is not due to a lack of competence, but a lack of nutrition.'

—ANONYMOUS

Today's women are a formidable force, adept at multitasking as they manage households, pursue careers and navigate various responsibilities. While their endeavours and priorities differ, self-care remains paramount. Neglecting self-care can lead to stress, impacting both menstrual and mental health. Chronic neglect can disrupt hormonal balance and lead to nutrient deficiencies, resulting in issues like painful cramps, excessive bleeding and even serious illnesses like cancer and type 2 diabetes.

There is no doubt that women are capable of achieving incredible success in diverse roles, whether as entrepreneurs, astronauts, educators, CEOs, volunteers or homemakers. However, it is essential to acknowledge that constant striving for the title of 'superwoman' can have detrimental effects on menstrual health. Women must prioritize self-care and follow a carefully structured routine of eating, sleeping, resting and working. This approach ensures that they maintain their physical and mental well-being, allowing them to thrive in their various roles without sacrificing their health.

Ultimately, it's crucial for women to recognize that their health, including menstrual health, is a priority that cannot be compromised. By prioritizing self-care, women can prevent hormonal imbalances, nutrient deficiencies and associated health concerns, and can continue to excel in their endeavours but also uphold optimal menstrual health and overall well-being.

FOCUS ON YOURSELF

Awareness: Early identification is key to addressing many health concerns. Monitoring bodily changes, understanding family history and recognizing lifestyle pressures can help us identify and treat disorders in their initial stages.

Physical exercise: Engaging in any form of movement is beneficial for both mind and body, whether through dedicated yoga practices, Pilates, mindful walking, swimming, cycling, participation in sports or regularly attending to daily chores. The World Health Organization (WHO) recommends 150 minutes of moderate to vigorous activity every week for adults aged 18–64 years.[104] While a regular fitness routine improves sleep quality, in contrast, excessive or faulty exercising can have negative consequences on our well-being.

Sleep: Adequate sleep is essential for rejuvenation and optimal functioning. In our fast-paced world, neglecting proper sleep deprives our bodies of their habitual repair and regeneration, thereby increasing cortisol levels (stress hormones). Establishing a regular sleep routine, aiming for 6–8 hours of deep sleep, supports overall health and disease prevention.

[104] 'Physical Activity', *World Health Organization*, 5 October 2022, https://www.who.int/news-room/fact-sheets/detail/physical-activity.

Sleep variations can also occur based on individual *doshas* and hormonal fluctuations.

Food: Nutrition plays a fundamental role in maintaining health. Fresh, natural, organic and home-cooked foods are essential for optimal well-being. Nutrients present in whole grains, nuts, healthy fats and fruits and vegetables, with most of them having a limited shelf life as nature intended, are most beneficial for us. Food preserved in the refrigerator and reheated can satisfy only the taste buds but often lacks essential nutrients.

Despite mindful eating based on the needs of our cycles, we may still be deprived of essential nutrients, which may be due to adulterated, genetically modified, pesticide-laden food or wrong pairings that may go against our body's constitution. Stress eating or not eating on time are some of the factors that have proved to be counterproductive. The foods we consume greatly impact our gut health and the quality of our sleep.

Macro and micronutrients: Macro and micronutrients are essential components of all foods, providing the body with the necessary elements for optimal functioning. Macronutrients are fats, carbohydrates and proteins required by the body in large quantities, while micronutrients such as vitamins and minerals are commonly found in fibre-rich fruits and vegetables and are required in smaller proportions (<100 mg/day).[105] Both these vital nutrients are found in a variety of food items, play a critical role in maintaining health and are identified as Vitamins A, B, C, D, E and K; as well as calcium; magnesium; potassium; iron; zinc; and selenium. Water is also an essential micronutrient.

[105]Venkatesh, U., Akash Sharma, Velmurugan A. Ananthan, Padmavathi Subbiah, R. Durga, and CSIR Summer Research Training Team, 'Micronutrient's Deficiency in India: A Systematic Review and Meta-analysis,' Vol. 10, 2021, e110. https://doi.org/10.1017%2Fjns.2021.102.

Supplements: Experts opine that modern food is inadequate in providing essential nutrients due to factors like depleted soil, pesticide use and nutrient loss during preservation and transportation.[106] These deficiencies become the culprits for underlying health conditions in the long run, resulting in researchers advocating the use of natural plant-derived supplements to replenish our bodies with the missing nutrients.[107] However, it is crucial to use these supplements under medical guidance to ensure safety and efficacy in boosting energy, immunity and bone health and preventing chronic ailments.

Natural, herbal and Ayurvedic supplements can be beneficial to women and can address almost all issues. However, it is important to ensure they are ethically sourced and of high quality. Factors such as expiration date, manufacturing practices and product authenticity should be considered when choosing supplements. Consulting with a qualified healthcare professional or nutritionist can help individuals make informed decisions about supplement use to support overall health and well-being.

THE ESSENTIALS

'Be good to yourself. If you don't take care of your body, where will you live?'

—KOBI YAMADA

Our ancestors consumed naturally grown local food, fruits and vegetables without chemical or pesticide treatments. Food was grown seasonally and had all the essential nutrients for

[106]Lovell, Rachel, 'How Modern Food Can Regain Its Nutrients,' *BBC*, https://www.bbc.com/future/bespoke/follow-the-food/why-modern-food-lost-its-nutrients/.

[107]Zebeaman, Meseret, Mesfin Getachew Tadesse, Rakesh Kumar Bachheti, Archana Bachheti, Rahel Gebeyhu, and Kundan Kumar Chaubey, 'Plants and Plant-derived Molecules as Natural Immunomodulators,' *Biomed Research International*, Vol. 2023, 2023, 7711297, https://doi.org/10.1155/2023/7711297.

sustenance. In the past, people relied on freshly ground oil, flour and spices to preserve the antioxidants and enzymes present in their food. However, in light of current circumstances, it is crucial to comprehend what we might be overlooking.

It is common knowledge that vitamins and minerals serve distinct purposes, and each person may derive varying benefits from different types of supplements. As a result, many women today require supplements tailored to their specific needs and deficiencies. Apart from dietary preferences such as vegetarian, vegan, eggetarian or non-vegetarian, it is essential to be mindful of one's age and take note of any underlying health concerns, long-term medication or allergies. Hence, self-medicating can prove to be counterproductive.

Women should take the initiative to educate themselves about their anatomy and recognize the importance of incorporating natural plant-based supplements into their routines. These supplements play a crucial role in maintaining menstrual regularity and providing support during pregnancy, childbirth and menopause. However, it is imperative that we also identify the potential benefits and drawbacks of specific supplement varieties. In her book *What You Must Know About Vitamins, Minerals, Herbs & More,* Pamela Wartian Smith, MD, MPH, delves into strategies for maintaining health and reversing diseases by harnessing the power of nutrients.[108]

Micronutrients are vital for the body to resist infections, stabilize the nervous system and aid in healing and restoring the body. Sometimes the required amount of micronutrients cannot be obtained from a regular diet.

This shortfall may stem from a weakened gut incapable of absorbing sufficient nutrients from food or from the poor

[108]Smith, Pamela Wartian, *What You Must Know About Vitamins, Minerals, Herbs & More: Choosing the Nutrients That Are Right for You,* Square One, New York, NY, 15 September 2007.

quality of available food resources or perhaps a combination of both factors. Regardless, replenishing the body with supplements has become the need of the hour and we must educate ourselves on its proper usage.

The demand for supplements has led to a multitude of companies flooding the market with Ayurvedic/herbal or super green supplements, each coming in different combinations and formulae, with recommended dosages, and promising to help restore lost nutrients.

The following micronutrients are essential for every woman's menstrual, physical and emotional health (the dosage can vary):

Iron (10 mg per day)

If you have been feeling exhausted lately and find it challenging to climb stairs without getting winded, despite being physically fit, these symptoms could indicate a lack of iron. Iron is a mineral essential for facilitating oxygen flow throughout the body and is needed to support immune functions and improve moods, memory and metabolism.

Iron deficiency is particularly common in women due to menstrual bleeding and the physiological demands of pregnancy, including potential abortions, which can result in low haemoglobin levels and anaemia. As a result, it is crucial for women to regularly monitor and replenish their iron levels. In contrast, men typically store more iron in their bodies.[109]

A dosage of 10 mg is normally advised to be taken in the mornings one hour after breakfast. Taking an iron supplement along with Vitamin C helps in the better absorption of this mineral.

[109]Eberts, Dan, 'How Much Iron Do Men Need Daily?,' *OneBlood*, 2 July 2019, https://www.oneblood.org/blog/how-much-iron-do-men-need-daily.html.

Natural sources of iron are green leafy vegetables, spinach, legumes, seeds, kidney beans, peas, whole grain, flax seeds, hemp seeds, pumpkin seeds, sesame seeds, raisins, pomegranates, bananas, prunes, citrus fruits and melons.

Vitamin B12 (1–2 mg per day)

If you are suffering from insomnia or sleep-related problems and experiencing low energy levels, it might be time to get your B12 levels checked. This important nutrient plays a critical role in supporting proper brain, nerve and cardiovascular functioning, thereby improving mental and physical energy. Vitamin B12 is normally paired with folate because each depends on the other for proper absorption and functioning. Vitamins can enhance brain regulation and developmental processes and prevent damage to neurons. Thus, it is vital to regularly monitor their levels.

Water-soluble vitamins like B12 are best taken in the morning on an empty stomach with a glass of water.

Natural sources include aloe vera juice; grass-fed, desi cow's milk and dairy products; free-range, organic, whole eggs; chia seeds; shiitake mushrooms; non-fat Greek yoghurt; nutritional yeast; tuna; and salmon.

Biotin (30 mcg per day)

If you are experiencing thinning of hair lately, along with dry, sallow and dehydrated skin or if your hair is losing its sheen, it may be worth getting your biotin (Vitamin B7) levels tested. Biotin is responsible for the healthy functioning of the brain and amino acid metabolism. It strengthens and improves the lustre of hair and nails, along with boosting the skin's health and vitality.

The best time for a biotin supplement is in the mornings on an empty stomach, or it can be taken an hour after meals with a glass of water.

Natural sources of biotin are present in organic nuts such as peanuts and walnuts, nut butter, whole grain and cereals, bananas, eggs and cauliflower.

Magnesium (350 mg per day)

If you are someone who frequently complains about headaches and gets nervous easily or feels that your nails and bones are getting brittle, then these issues may be due to low magnesium levels in the body. Magnesium is a vital mineral that is a co-factor in over 300 enzyme systems in our bodies that are responsible for diverse biochemical reactions.[110] It assists and supports cardiovascular health and promotes positive thoughts, thereby reducing PMS symptoms. It is also responsible for increasing muscle strength and preventing bloating, water retention and cramps. It is most effective when taken after meals.

Natural sources of magnesium include almonds, spinach, roasted cashews, oil-roasted peanuts, soy milk, organic legumes, black/kidney beans, chickpeas, avocado, banana, potatoes with skin, cabbage, beans, figs and seeds.

Calcium (1000 mg per day)

If you recently stumbled on something and wondered how you ended up with a fracture, or suffer from osteoporosis or other bone-related problems, or unexpectedly gained a lot of weight, or are in your post-menopausal stage, then you may be in need of calcium supplements. Calcium is responsible for the proper functioning of the heart, a strong nervous and muscular system and for building and maintaining the strength of teeth and bones.

These supplements are best taken along with food and in

[110]Faryadi, Qais, 'The Magnificent Effect of Magnesium to Human Health: A Critical Review', 2012, https://www.researchgate.net/publication/266869482_The_Magnificent_Effect_of_Magnesium_to_Human_Health_A_Critical_Review.

doses not exceeding 500-600 mg at a time. Iron and calcium supplements should not be taken simultaneously, as each group can interfere with the absorption of the other. Calcium works well with Biotin as both are important for healthy hair and nails.

Natural sources of calcium include broccoli, kale, oranges, figs, organic dairy products (A2 milk, butter, ghee, yoghurt, cheese), tofu, soy products, Brazil nuts, almonds, papaya and pineapple.

Vitamin D3 (15 mcg per day) or 1,500-2,000 IU per day

If you frequently experience body/muscle aches, inertia and lethargy and often suffer from cough and cold, then your Vitamin D levels need to be tested. Also known as the 'sunshine vitamin,' it is naturally produced in the skin in response to sunlight.

This vitamin builds strong bones by helping the body absorb calcium. It supports the immune system, sets up a strong muscle network, fights depression, increases fertility rate and also affects the way each cell carries out its function. It has powerful antioxidant and anti-inflammatory effects, delays brain degeneration and increases cognitive functions.

This supplement is best taken during the first half of the day with a breakfast that contains healthy fats for proper absorption. It can be paired with calcium or other supplements for easy absorption.

Natural sources of Vitamin D3 include sunlight, organic cereals, tofu, fatty fish sardines, mackerel, egg yolks, shiitake mushrooms, desi cow milk and oatmeal.

Maintaining optimum levels of micronutrients through supplements may seem enticing but they should not be viewed as alternatives to meals. Instead, they should be seen only as enhancers for nutrients and not as substitutes for nutritious food. While a well-balanced diet of macro and micronutrients is essential, it doesn't always guarantee optimal health. Hence, consulting a trusted nutritionist is highly recommended for personalized guidance on dietary needs and supplement usage.

AYURVEDA TO THE RESCUE

'The doctor of the future will give no medication,
but will interest his patients in
the care of the human frame, diet
and in the cause and prevention of disease.'

—THOMAS A. EDISON

Ayurveda embraces a holistic perspective that integrates nutrition, physical activity and lifestyle modifications with the utilization of herbal supplements for healing. With a rich history dating back thousands of years, this science of longevity promotes wellness through a variety of plants, fruits, roots and herbs as medicines.

Backed by science, certain Ayurvedic herbal medicines possess potent and efficient curative properties, contributing to overall health when administered properly. As an avid follower of Ayurveda and having personally reaped the benefits of these herbs, I aim to introduce some popular and effective herbs along with their recommended dosage.[111] This information is only for a common understanding of their properties and benefits, and not meant for self-medication. Even Ayurvedic medicines or herbal supplements do have side effects if prescribed without considering factors such as the proper ratio, body constitution

[111] '8 Powerful Ayurvedic Herbs with Their Great Benefits', *PharmEasy*, 4 January 2024, https://pharmeasy.in/blog/8-powerful-ayurvedic-herbs-with-their-great-benefits/.

or the prevailing health conditions. Consulting with a qualified practitioner or herbalist provides valuable guidance tailored to individual needs and circumstances.

Shatavari

Also known as the 'Queen of Herbs,' Shatavari acts as a rejuvenating tonic for women due to its immense support to the reproductive system. It aids in balancing heavy flow and lubricating vaginal dryness. This species of the asparagus plant is considered a staple in Ayurvedic medicine for its anti-ageing, anti-inflammatory and antioxidant properties. Additionally, it supports the immune, cognitive and digestive functions, while also helping to prevent physical and emotional stress.

Dosage: One-fourth teaspoon of the tonic with milk or honey twice a day after lunch and dinner, or as advised by the medical practitioner. It is available both in tablet and capsule form.

Ashwagandha

This popular herb, also known as Indian ginseng, is indeed a 'magic potion' for women of all ages. It is renowned in Ayurvedic medicine due to its competence in fighting infection, promoting sound sleep and boosting memory. It is a woman's best aid in managing PMS symptoms and reproductive hormones. It acts as an effective stress reliever, significantly reducing cortisol levels.

Dosage: 250–500 mg per day with milk at night or as advised by an Ayurvedic practitioner.

Triphala

Triphala is a staple in almost every Indian household. Triphala's usage can be dated back to thousands of years for its healing properties. It is a combination of three fruits—amla, bibhitaki and haritaki. It acts as a multipurpose treatment for various symptoms, including digestive issues, inflammations, weight loss and dental cavities. It is commonly used for treating constipation.

Dosage: Half a teaspoon mixed with warm water or ghee and honey before bedtime.

Ashoka

Ashoka, meaning 'no grief' in Sanskrit, is revered as one of the most sacred trees in Hindu tradition. In Indian mythology, it is dedicated to the 'God of Love' Kama because of its women-friendly properties of regulating menstrual flow, balancing hormones, treating reproductive disorders, toning and healing the womb and easing cramps, along with improving skin health.

Dosage: Taking 2–3 ml with the same measure of water after lunch and dinner can help in controlling heavy menstrual bleeding. The dosage may be adjusted by the practitioner based on individual requirements.

Nettle

Nettle serves as a natural multivitamin, rich in nutrients, minerals and iron. Deeply nourishing for the pre- and post-menstrual cycle, fertility and postpartum care and assists the body in healing after a miscarriage.

Dosage: One capsule daily with water with lunch or dinner.

Neem

Neem leaf powder is used to balance the pitta and kapha doshas and treat vata disorders, making it an essential component of Ayurvedic medicine. It serves as an excellent pain reliever and its blood-purifying properties help in curing acne and rashes.

Neem flushes out toxins, cures ulcers and is good for skin and hair.

Dosage: One tablet twice a day, before lunch and dinner, along with a glass of warm water. Dosage can vary depending on individual needs.

SEED CYCLING

Seed cycling is the natural method of balancing hormones using seeds.[112] While you are weighing the advantages of herbal supplements, let me introduce you to seed cycling, a widely tried-and-tested way of balancing hormones. It simply involves selectively rotating four different types of seeds in your diet—flax, pumpkin, sesame and sunflower seeds—based on the body's requirements during the four phases of the menstrual cycle. Seed cycling is gaining popularity due to negligible side effects, simple usage and proven effectiveness.

Dr Lindsey Jesswein was the first to come up with a modern seed-cycling method.[113] This nutrition-based approach then became popular among some women as these seeds have natural oestrogen and progesterone boosting properties, along with certain oils and nutrients that help to balance hormones. These mini superfoods are a rich source of healthy fatty acids, vitamins, minerals, antioxidants, phytoestrogens and a type of fibre called lignin that is good for female hormones. As these seeds are all in concentrated forms, just a tablespoon of seeds every day is sufficient for healthy menstrual cycles.

[112]Vidushi, 'Seed Cycling for Balanced Hormones', *Sprig & Vine*, 22 January 2019, http://sprigandvine.in/seed-cycling/.

[113]'Seed Cycling for Natural Hormonal Balance', *Dr Lindsey Jesswein, ND*, 17 March 2017, https://www.drlindseynd.com/blog/seed-cycling-for-natural-hormonal-balance.

KNOW YOUR SUPER SEEDS

Flax seeds: They contain phytoestrogens (natural, plant-based compounds) and omega-3 fatty acids, which promote blood flow to the uterus, reduce inflammation and promote digestive health. They are also high in lignans that help control excess oestrogen and reduce PMS symptoms.

Pumpkin seeds: They are rich in zinc and omega-3 fatty acids, which support progesterone secretion, and control progesterone deficiency symptoms like migraines, depression, anxiety and mood swings, especially during the second phase of the menstrual cycle.

Sesame seeds: They contain lignan, which regulates excess oestrogen and encourages progesterone production. They are high in zinc and Omega-6 fatty acids, boost fertility and help manage PMS symptoms.

Sunflower seeds: They are high in selenium, which balances hormones and aids detoxification of the liver along with boosting healthy functioning. These seeds are also loaded with Vitamin E, which supports progesterone secretion during the luteal phase. They are also high in the essential omega-6 fatty acids and magnesium, which are good for decreasing muscle tension and are required for strong bones, respectively.

CYCLE SYNCING

Synchronising the seed cycle with the menstrual cycle is the art of balancing your hormones with specific nutrients.[114] Let me

[114]'Cycle Syncing 101: A Beginner's Guide to Holistically Rebalancing Your Hormones', *Dr. Will Cole, IFMCP, DNM, DC,* Cole Natural Health Centers, LLC, https://drwillcole.com/hormone-health/cycle-syncing-101-a-beginners-guide-to-holistically-rebalancing-your-hormones.

shed some light on the need for selected seeds during specific menstrual phases, along with their nutritional values, as they can help make positive menstruation a reality.

Days 1–13 (Menstrual to Follicular Phases)

Seeds: Flax and Pumpkin

1. Begin Phase 1 of seed cycling by consuming 1 tbsp of ground flaxseeds and 1 tbsp of pumpkin seeds each day, from the first day of menstruation until the next 13 days.
2. Both flax and pumpkin seeds help in increasing oestrogen levels and improving ovulation for healthy egg production.
3. Lignans in flaxseed block excess oestrogen secretion while zinc-rich pumpkin seeds help to support progesterone levels, which transpire in the next phase.

Days 14–28 (Ovulatory to Luteal Phases)

Seeds: Sesame and Sunflower

1. Begin Phase 2 of seed cycling by consuming 1 tbsp of sunflower seeds and 1 tbsp of sesame seeds, from Day 14 to Day 28 or until menstruation begins.
2. The main objective of ingesting both these seeds during this phase is to boost progesterone levels and also to strengthen the liver.
3. Sunflower seeds, high in Vitamin E and selenium, help regulate excess oestrogen, while sesame seeds, rich in zinc and selenium, tone and strengthen the uterus. Both these seeds contain lignans, which are necessary to regulate hormones.

Some women do not have the benefit of a regular 28-day cycle. However, they can still follow seed cycling by dividing their own personal periodic cycle equally and commencing from the day of their period. These seeds may be consumed at any time of the day, either whole or ground, or as inclusions in smoothies, porridge, rotis and healthy snacks.

Buying natural, organic, whole and unsalted seeds is as important as their consumption. They can be refrigerated and used in small quantities to maintain their freshness. Overnight soaking in water helps in easy digestion. One can also include soaked chia, peanuts or almonds, along with the cycling seeds for added nutrition. A great advantage of these seeds is that they are rich in fibre, protein, calcium and various healthy nutrients and the good fat present in them is essential to balance the hormones.

However, despite their multiple benefits, it is always advisable to exercise caution and be aware of any allergies or discomforts before eating nuts or seeds. Maintaining a journal can help to keep track of daily symptoms.

Be patient and consistent as these seeds take time to work on the body. Missing a day or two is also completely fine. The positive changes take time but are enough to inspire one to continue this intake as part of a healthy diet. Believe in it to experience the difference.

THE BOTTOM LINE

Choosing a diet made of nutrient-rich foods is vital despite the emphasis on vitamins and mineral supplements. Supplements contain necessary vitamins and minerals with few calories but a healthy diet nourishes the body and provides the right amount of energy to meet daily needs. Making necessary modifications in your dietary habits and sleep patterns and adopting exercise and breathing techniques along with the right supplements are the mantras that can unfold the secret to great health.

NIMMI'S MANTRA

Life operates in a synchronized manner and it is our responsibility to align with it and take action.

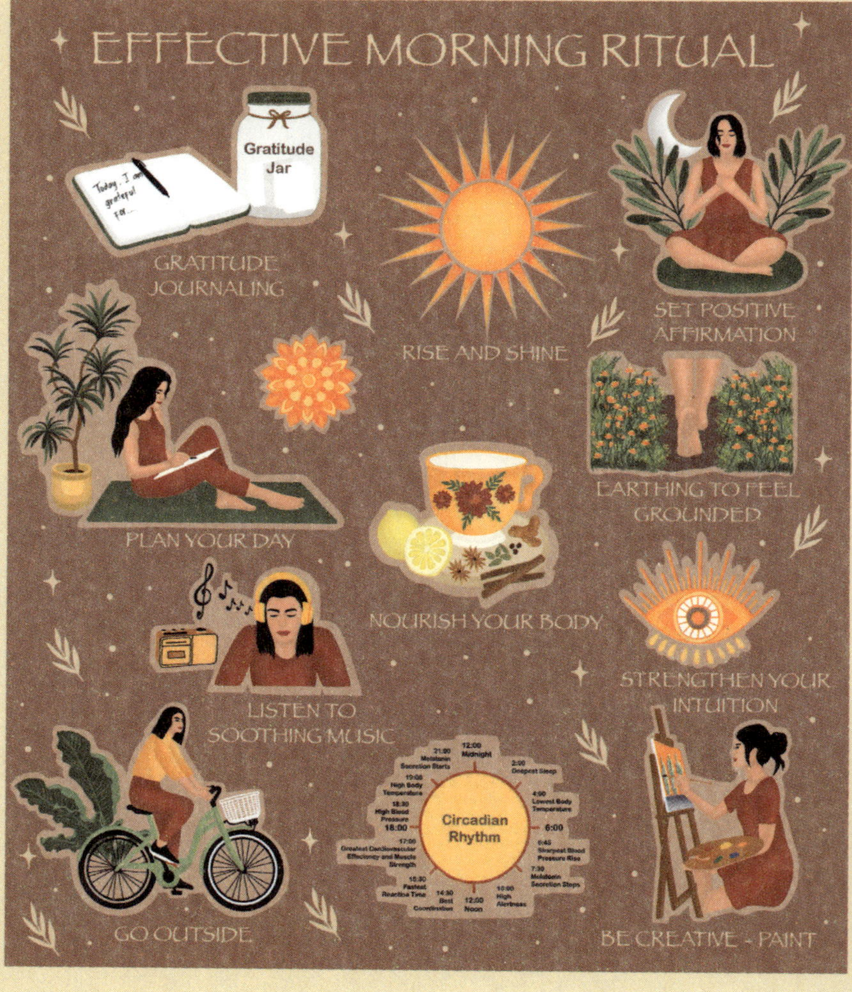
EFFECTIVE MORNING RITUAL
Today, I am grateful for...
Gratitude Jar
GRATITUDE JOURNALING
RISE AND SHINE
SET POSITIVE AFFIRMATION
PLAN YOUR DAY
EARTHING TO FEEL GROUNDED
NOURISH YOUR BODY
LISTEN TO SOOTHING MUSIC
STRENGTHEN YOUR INTUITION
Circadian Rhythm
12:00 Midnight
2:00 Deepest Sleep
4:00 Lowest Body Temperature
6:00
6:45 Sharpest Blood Pressure Rise
7:30 Melatonin Secretion Stops
10:00 High Alertness
12:00 Noon
14:30 Best Coordination
15:30 Fastest Reaction Time
17:00 Greatest Cardiovascular Efficiency and Muscle Strength
18:00
18:30 High Blood Pressure
19:00 High Body Temperature
21:00 Melatonin Secretion Starts
GO OUTSIDE
BE CREATIVE - PAINT

12

MINDFUL MORNINGS

'Success is nothing more than a few simple disciplines, practised every day.'

—JIM ROHN

In this era of digitalization, humans are gradually falling out of sync with nature. We work at night, sleep during the day, eat during hours meant for rest and hide from sunlight by living under artificial lights. These habits may genuinely be due to unavoidable commitments, physical ailments, medication or monetary necessities but their harmful effects eventually become detrimental to health and lower the quality of life.

A healthy *dinacharya* (daily routine) is essential to promote the practice of self-care through daily activities. Self-care begins with an effective morning ritual, as detailed in this chapter.

OUR INNER BODY CLOCK

Before delving into an effective morning routine, let us discuss the importance and relevance of the internal body clock, also known as the circadian rhythm. This rhythm entails the subtle change that occurs in the body over a 24-hour period, with approximately 16 hours of wakefulness and 8 hours of sleep at night. The circadian rhythm is influenced by light and darkness, among other factors. These bio-rhythmic activities are controlled by the hypothalamus in the brain and receive direct input from the eyes. It is purely nature-ordained, not only in humans but in all types of species for their well-being.

A night of restful, high-quality sleep can significantly enhance both physical and mental performance the following day. This remarkable improvement occurs as the brain releases serotonin, which serves as a vital messenger, transmitting signals between nerve cells in the brain and the rest of the body. When exposed to morning sunlight, this mood-enhancing hormone acts as a stabilizer, keeping you alert and focused throughout the day.

The modern world, with its insatiable demand for productivity and profit, is indiscriminately imposing unreasonable work schedules upon the current generation, disregarding the natural rhythms of the human body. This has resulted in people being glued to technology and feeling disconnected from the body's natural sleep-wake cycle. Consequently, individuals are forced to subsist in survival mode, eating and sleeping at unnatural hours to comply with their company's demands.

Women in particular are vulnerable to the consequences of a disrupted circadian rhythm, as hormonal fluctuations can severely weaken their immunity. Prolonged periods of sedentary work and inadequate nutrition only exacerbate the pressure on the reproductive system. This can lead to a rise in menstrual and mental health issues. Recognizing the critical role of sleep, women must cultivate a robust morning routine to promote optimal health. It is also important to wake up at the same time every day, including on weekends.[115]

[115]Panda, Satchin, *The Circadian Code*, Vermilion, London, 28 June 2018.

AYURVEDIC MORNINGS

The cornerstone of a prosperous future rests in steadfast adherence to a nourishing daily routine. Crafting a potent morning ritual holds the power to fortify the body, mind and spirit. By emphasizing the regularity of a balanced lifestyle, women can harmonize their internal energies, overcome gut imbalances and enhance nutrient absorption. A typical daily routine may include:

1. *Rise and Shine*

Awaken with the morning sun and bask in its yellow glow as it invigorates the body with serotonin. This natural mood booster imbues the mind with unyielding willpower, laser-sharp focus and invigorating motivation, fostering overall well-being. It inspires the body to arise without the need for alarms.

- Rising at the same time every day stabilizes cortisol (stress hormone) levels, thereby bringing full vitality to the body.
- Touch the ground barefoot, sit up to take a few deep breaths and awaken all your senses with gratitude.
- A clean bed declutters the mind instantly and awakens a sense of accomplishment. It also sets a pattern in the brain for sound sleep the following night.
- Strengthen your in-built connection with the Earth (also known as earthing or grounding) by walking barefoot for 10–15 minutes every day. The idea is that our bodies, through direct contact, absorb the free electrons, which act as antioxidants and strengthen our immunity levels.[116]

[116]Kinch, Georgia, 'Body-Earthing,' *The Ohio State University*, 18 April 2018, https://u.osu.edu/vanzandt/2018/04/18/body-earthing/.

2. *The Hygiene Ritual*

- Revitalize your senses and invigorate the mind by splashing water on your face. Multiple splashes are recommended for optimal rejuvenation. In today's gadget-infused world, staring at the screen for too long can strain our eyes and cause dryness and fatigue as these devices emit blue light, which is the main reason for vision problems. Preserve your eye health by cleansing your eyes daily with a DIY solution (by soaking organic rose petals in warm water overnight).
- Maintain oral hygiene by mindfully brushing your teeth with soft and natural bristles, using herbal paste or powder with neem extracts. Bitter herbs have potent, antibacterial properties beneficial for oral hygiene. Massaging the gums is an important ritual to hold the teeth together. Regular tongue scraping could help remove bacterial deposits and foul smells, along with improving the sensitivity of taste buds, by stimulating digestive fire (agni).

3. *The Art of Drinking Water*

Practice the art of drinking water (*Usha paana chikitsa*) to stay hydrated and healthy. Start your day by drinking at least 2–3 cups of warm water to flush out toxins from the intestine. Water stored in a copper, silver or glass vessel can be beneficial to your body. Savour the water slowly and mindfully, in small sips, while sitting comfortably with a straight back to strengthen your digestive system. Water has the power to balance all three doshas and promote holistic wellness. Avoid consuming too cold or packaged water as it lacks life force (prana).

- This therapeutic ritual of drinking water in the morning energizes 100 trillion cells, activates all the internal organs, flushes out toxins through the kidneys, raises the body's temperature and speeds up metabolism. It also helps to prevent ailments.

- Most importantly, abstain from starting the day with coffee or tea on an empty stomach as it can affect your gut microbiome. Instead, you may have a beverage only after consuming a few glasses of water.

4. *The Elimination Process*

Clearing the bladder in the morning flushes out accumulated toxins.

- Bowel elimination can be initiated by drinking plain water followed by a warm, herbal or Ayurvedic concoction that helps in the smooth clearing of the bowels.
- Developing a morning routine can prevent constipation.
- Triphala is a popular Ayurvedic *churna* (powder), which when taken with warm water before bedtime can help maintain a routine.
- Watch out for the colour and smell of urine and stool as it says a lot about your eating habits and health.
- Squatting on the toilet, as against sitting on today's western toilets, puts less strain on the rectal canal and prevents serious issues such as haemorrhoids and pelvic prolapses.
- Your food intake, lack of sleep, stress and anxieties at work can affect the elimination process. Hence, care should be taken to include fibre-rich food in all three meals of the day.

5. *Liver-friendly Drinks*

Including immunity-boosting health concoctions made with natural herbs and spices from your kitchen pharmacy in your diet can effectively fight disease-causing pathogens and strengthen the internal system.

- Drinking a glass of warm water mixed with a quarter of

a teaspoon of organic cinnamon powder, grated ginger, 1 tbsp of lemon juice, honey and a pinch of pink salt makes for a rejuvenating drink. Ginger helps with digestion and boosts immunity. Cinnamon has antiviral properties and regulates blood sugar. Lemon reduces inflammation by cleansing harmful bacteria. These ingredients make this a perfect liver-boosting tonic and can be altered to suit an individual body's requirements.

Other options that you can consider are:

- Incorporating a daily ritual of soaking half a teaspoon of organic fenugreek seeds overnight and consuming both the seeds and the water on an empty stomach alleviates digestive issues, curbs bloating and aids in weight management.
- Consuming raisins soaked overnight first thing in the morning, before having any other food, can act as a natural laxative. It also rids the body of toxins and purifies the blood.

6. *Early Morning Walks*

Taking a leisurely morning walk in nature can be an effective way to refresh your mind and boost creativity. Surround yourself with the symphony of natural sounds of nature, such as the gentle rustle of leaves, the whistling wind, the melodious chirping of birds and the cool breeze on your face. These experiences can elevate your mood and help to clear your mind. Furthermore, exposure to natural light and green spaces has been scientifically proven to boost serotonin levels, reduce anxiety, regulate mood and increase energy. A peaceful and quiet morning enables a deeper appreciation of the world and contributes to long-term good health.

7. Move Your Body

In the mornings when kapha dosha predominates is the best time for fluid body movements. Choose a sustainable and enjoyable exercise regime, such as performing sun salutations (*surya namaskar*), rhythmic yoga stretches, dance sequences, leisurely swimming or cycling. All these activities bring an adrenaline rush to the body without inducing exhaustion. Most importantly, maintaining consistency in these health regimes enhances flexibility, naturally lubricating the joints and relieving stress. Consistently engaging in an exercise regime also makes us feel proud and accomplished.

8. Self-massage and Bathing Ritual

After the exertions mentioned above, the body has now developed a healthy sheen of sweat, signalling the right time for a few minutes of rejuvenation through massage. A quick self-massage (dry-brush or oil massage) offers preventive and curative health benefits, especially when followed as a daily routine.

- Begin by rubbing a few drops of organic, cold-pressed sesame oil (for the vata and kapha body types), or coconut or Mahanarayana Ayurvedic oil (for a pitta body) into your palms for a minute to generate warmth. Gently massage this warm oil, starting from the feet, and gradually moving upwards, towards the heart. This method effectively stimulates blood circulation and detoxifies the body.
- A bath serves as an excellent means to cleanse one's aura or energetic field. Follow it with a shower of warm or tepid water, depending on the prevailing season, to feel fresh throughout the day. Cold showers naturally stimulate the Vagus nerve, which is closely connected to the brain and

the heart.[117] While under the water, visualize all negative thoughts and energy being washed away.

- Cleanse and nourish the skin using organic scrubs, which effectively remove dead skin and excess oil while alleviating feelings of fatigue.

9. *Pranayama: The Art of Breathing*

Now that the body is feeling invigorated after a refreshing bath, it is time to focus on your breathing to cleanse the mind. Pranayama plays a significant role in promoting mental health by reducing anxiety and overthinking while improving concentration. It is a breathing technique to strengthen the connection between the mind and body for renewed energy.

- Sitting quietly in a comfortable position, either on a chair or a mat, keeping the spine straight, brings coherence to thoughts and emotions.
- With closed eyes, inhale and exhale deeply for a few minutes consciously. Observe your breath flowing in and out, ensuring that the stomach and chest expand and contract rhythmically.
- Pranayama encompasses various breathing techniques that should be practised under expert guidance. For instance, a pitta person can follow Sheetali, a kapha person benefits from Bhastrika, while a vata person benefits more from Nadi Shodhana pranayama.
- A suitable breathing programme is essential for coping with anxiety, depression and loneliness, and also demanding work, fatigue and maintaining healthy boundaries and

[117]'Cold Showers to Activate Your Vagus Nerve and Calm Parasympathetic System,' *Trudy Scott*, 5 October 2020, https://www.everywomanover29.com/blog/cold-showers-to-activate-your-vagus-nerve-and-calm-parasympathetic-system-26-other-anxiety-busting-tips/.

expectations. Practicing deep breathing even for a few minutes every day can clear physical and emotional blocks, making it easier to navigate life's challenges.

- This spiritual practice (sadhana) can purify all 72,000 channels (*nadis*) in the body by increasing blood circulation, boosting sleep, prompting a healthy appetite, strengthening immunity and building mental performance, thereby helping in stress management.

10. *Mindful Meditation*

After energizing the body with personalized breathing techniques, dedicate the next 15 minutes of your daily routine to meditation.

- Everything in life is an experience. While some experiences are gained through actions and others through expressions, meditation is experienced through introspection. Meditation serves as a stepping stone towards your goals and maintains a consistent balance between your body, mind and soul.
- Mindfulness is the art of being present in the moment. This can happen by unleashing the natural workings of the mind and allowing thoughts to pass as they arise by suspending undue judgements.
- Begin meditating for five minutes initially and gradually progress for longer durations based on your daily schedule. It is natural to lose focus, and if the mind wanders, simply redirect your focus to your breath.
- Consider meditation as a commitment to reconnect with yourself. Make use of any of the innumerable meditation apps or videos that are available for beginners to get through the initial period of distraction.
- Morning meditation helps the body and mind to focus on the present moment. Allow this positive energy to flow within

the body, enhancing the ability to manage relationships and creating more compassion towards the self and others.

Meditation acts as a natural stimulant, illuminating your thinking power and motivating you to be a part of solutions. Make the most of its manifold benefits by incorporating it into your routine consistently.

11. *Gratitude Journaling*

Incorporate gratitude journaling into your daily morning routine by jotting down the following affirmations:

- I am overflowing with gratitude for the gift of life.
- I am deeply thankful for the countless blessings in my life.
- I have unwavering faith in my intuition to make wise decisions.
- I possess everything required to triumph today.
- I am overflowing with kindness, affection and generosity.

This morning ritual of gratitude journaling cultivates not only personal advancement but also spiritual awareness. By reflecting on our graces, we process our emotions and enhance our well-being. These powerful affirmations provide a dynamic and optimistic launch pad for the day ahead. To amplify the impact of this ritual, end it by rubbing your palms together. This action activates the electromagnetic energy in your body and opens your mind to the limitless possibilities of the day ahead.[118]

12. *Nourishing Food*

With almost all the morning self-care activities completed, you have truly earned your breakfast. The most important ritual of

---

[118]Harrison, Theo, 'Understanding the Seven Layers of the Human Aura: Their Functions and Meanings,' *Mind Journal*, https://themindsjournal.com/layers-of-human-aura/.

the day is to fuel your body with nutritious food and charge it for the day.

- Food savoured with gratitude becomes the building blocks of bodily tissue.
- Breakfast should replenish the supply of glucose to boost energy levels and provide all essential nutrients required for the sustenance of the body.
- It is recommended to have an early breakfast that is light, nutritious and healthy, ideally taken before 10.30 a.m.
- Boost your mood by consuming fruit or vegetable smoothies. They should preferably be had half an hour before breakfast as the stomach needs time to assimilate them. Moreover, including a variety of fruits and vegetables ensures that you're getting a wide range of vitamins, minerals and antioxidants, which can contribute to better health.
- Opt for a traditional, local and nutritious breakfast such as dosa, idli, parathas, poha, upma, healthy pancakes or other options like soaked overnight oats, warm porridge with jaggery or a bowl of savoury oats seasoned with spices and nuts. These options offer ample protein, healthy fats and fibre.
- Some people prefer a spicy or salty breakfast while others crave sweeter versions. It is important to monitor your energy levels mid-morning and adjust your breakfast choices accordingly. Your breakfast should act as a brain booster, sustaining you until lunchtime.
- If you need a boost between meals, consider homemade energy bars with nuts and seeds, or snack on fresh fruit or medjool dates. These snacks are rich in natural sugars and fibres, providing sustained energy and preventing hunger pangs.
- Cold food or milkshakes can dampen the gut fire (agni) and are best avoided.

13. *Digital Detox*

It is vital to refrain from social media right in the morning. It has a way of unduly dragging minds into others' activities. Be mindful of the energy you set for the day by using it for productive purposes and prioritize your own day's activities. Avoid mindless scrolling for greater mental health and peace as it can lead the mind astray and cause anxiety.

14. *Evening Rituals*

Preparing for a better morning begins the night before. Therefore, it is crucial to adopt a calming evening routine that allows both the mind and body to unwind and prepare for restful sleep. Avoid low-energy foods, typically processed ones like refined sugars and unhealthy fats, which can prevent feelings of lethargy and imbalance in the body. Additionally, refrain from engaging in intense discussions, watching violent or negative content, horror films or discussing heavy topics like loss, death or relationship problems after dusk. Similarly, avoid listening to stimulating music genres like heavy metal or pop, as they can negatively impact the brain and disrupt sleep patterns, leading to increased stress and anxiety. By limiting stimulating activities and nourishing oneself with fibre-rich nutrients, we can contribute to better sleep quality and wake up feeling refreshed for a brighter morning ahead.

Adequate sleep is essential to ensure that our minds and bodies are operating at their best. It is imperative to sleep for 6–8 hours each night in order to be fully alert and coherent during the day. The most rejuvenating period of sleep occurs between 10 p.m. and 2 a.m. during which the brain releases the hormone called melatonin that aids in the processes of fat burning, healing, repairing and restoring gut health.[119] Therefore, aiming to sleep by 10 p.m. every night, devoid of exposure to blue or artificial light, is crucial for maintaining the ultimate self-care routine.

Adopting a healthy self-care ritual is the most effortless way to tap the unlimited source of cosmic energy. It can accelerate the process of healing and reverse reproductive health issues.

THE BOTTOM LINE

Every decision taken in the morning can impact the subconscious and shape the outcome of the day. Prevention of disease begins with self-care and self-discipline. Regardless of background, self-care has to be seen as essential, not as a luxury. Effective morning rituals can help one live in harmony with nature and hormones.

NIMMI'S MANTRA

Leave the past behind, and let the future worry about itself. Today, take a deep breath and begin a new chapter in your life.

[119]'Why You Don't Want to Miss Out on Sleep Between 10 pm and 2 am', *Larissa Popp*, 8 August 2018, https://larissapopp.com/health-coaching/why-you-dont-want-to-miss-out-on-sleep-between-10pm-and-2am/.

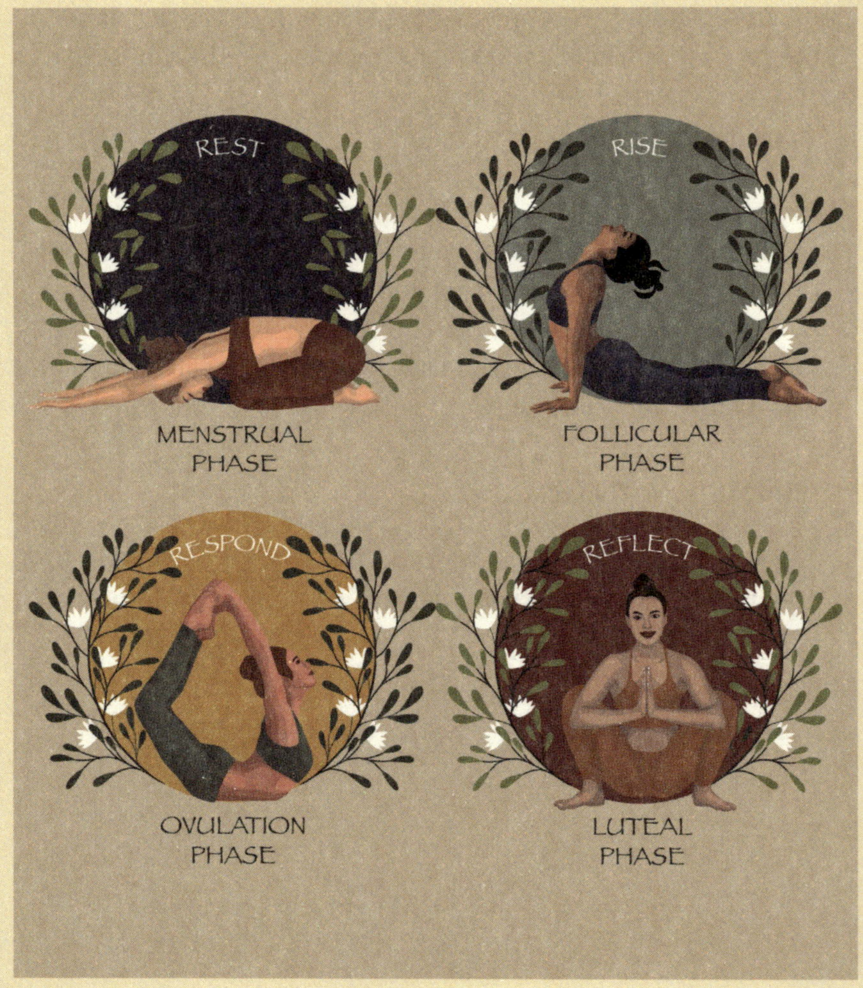
REST
MENSTRUAL PHASE
RISE
FOLLICULAR PHASE
RESPOND
OVULATION PHASE
REFLECT
LUTEAL PHASE

13

THE HOLISTIC POWER OF YOGA

'Yoga is a way to freedom. By its constant practice, we can free ourselves from fear, anguish and loneliness.'

—INDRA DEVI

Yoga, an ancient discipline originating in India over 5,000 years ago, is deeply intertwined with Ayurveda. The term 'yoga' in Sanskrit translates to the harmonious union of body and spirit.

Renowned yogi B.K.S. Iyengar famously remarked, 'Words cannot convey the value of yoga. It has to be experienced.'[120] To gain the full benefits of yoga, it's important to understand its three core components—*asanas* (body postures), pranayama (rhythmic breathing) and meditation (relaxing the mind)—and understand how they synergize to bring balance within the mind, body and spirit.

Yoga offers a holistic approach to well-being, seeking to establish a profound connection between the physical and emotional aspects of oneself. Its ultimate aim transcends mere physical fitness; it aims to attain peace and harmony between the mind, body and consciousness. Embracing yoga is a commitment towards achieving enduring tranquillity.

In essence, yoga encompasses the seamless integration of

[120]Iyengar, B.K.S., *B.K.S. Iyengar Yoga: The Path to Holistic Health*, Penguin USA, New York, NY, 23 December 2013.

graceful physical postures, the skilful mastery of breath control through pranayama and the exploration of in-depth meditation.

YOGA ASANAS

'The body is your temple.
Keep it pure and clean for the soul to reside in.'

—B.K.S. IYENGAR

The human body stands as a masterpiece of natural engineering, inherently designed for optimal movement and functions when engaged in activity. Yogic postures are known to integrate mental and physical realms through their rhythmic movements, fostering a sense of inner and outer balance. The focus of practice here depends not on intensity but on the sustainability that can support the body's natural cycles and hormonal balance.

A disciplined yoga regimen boosts the body's metabolic process, strengthens internal organs, improves the spine's alignment, tones muscles and lubricates the body's joints and ligaments. It also stimulates the reproductive glands and regularizes hormonal variations and menstrual flow. Establishing a sacred yoga routine is a tribute to your soul, unlocking enhanced flexibility, mobility, balance, clarity and strength.

CONSCIOUS BREATHING

'Every emotion is connected with the breath.
If you change the breath, change the rhythm,
you can change the emotion.'

—SRI SRI RAVI SHANKAR

Prana+Ayama means breath expansion. Pranayama is a practice of conscious or deliberate control over breathing to improve mental focus. Slow, rhythmic breathing strengthens the respiratory system and enriches the quality of blood. It calms the nervous system and helps in clearing emotional blockages, enabling the life force (prana) to move freely to permeate every cell and tissue. The power of your breath possesses the ability to influence the mood and course of your hormones.

MINDFUL MEDITATION

'Meditation is not a way of making your mind quiet.
It is a way of entering into the quiet that is already there.'

—DEEPAK CHOPRA

For centuries, Indian sages and Buddhist monks upheld the importance of meditation as a tool to focus the mind in order to strengthen intuitive power, which ultimately led them to attain wisdom. Meditation unveils the secrets of our soul, wisdom, healing and a deeper understanding of ourselves. This practice helps us to be mindful of the present by boosting our emotional quotient.

Meditation teaches us to appreciate the power of silence and embrace our deepest thoughts without judgment. Being mindful allows you to be creative and productive throughout the day, inducing a deep state of relaxation by channelling your energy in the right direction. Consistent practice orchestrates the regulation of hormonal fluctuations, granting us the gift of inner peace. It addresses our relentless anxiety and pervasive fear that lies at the root of modern stress, weaving a soothing symphony that harmonizes our inner world.

As a dedicated meditator for several decades, I can truly attest to the serenity that this practice has woven into the fabric of my life. Meditation has been my trusted guide on the path towards self-realization, revealing the multifaceted layers of my existence and unveiling my authentic self. In a world that ceaselessly beckons with distractions and constant hustle, meditation has been my sanctuary, providing moments of bliss and clarity.

GOOD AND BAD STRESS

Modern culture imposes a multitude of expectations and demands. It has brought into existence machines that require less physical work but produce more mental stress. Life is filled with a plethora of stressors, often overshadowing the importance of self-care amidst the pursuit of material success. Many women find themselves working tirelessly, pushing beyond their boundaries, which can lead to feelings of inadequacy, loneliness and anxiety, significantly impacting their reproductive health and vital hormones. Hence, it is crucial to follow circadian rhythms to ease the discomfort of the mind and the body.

Stress itself is neither inherently good nor bad; its impact depends on how it is managed. However, an optimum amount of positive stress, often called 'eustress,' is needed to keep the body motivated, focused and energized to accomplish tasks and achieve daily goals. Mild forms of acute stress enhance performance skills, strengthen survival instincts and also direct you to move ahead in life with optimism as the adrenaline glands release two hormones, adrenaline and cortisol to support the body's fight or flight mode.

Conversely, excessive or chronic distress is the hormonal response from the body, arising due to its inability to cope with various psychological and social issues. These stressors can activate the sympathetic nervous system, negatively affecting both physical and mental well-being. Examples include procrastination, work pressure, stress from deadlines and targets, inability to deal with colleagues or superiors, chemical addictions of all kinds, inability to manage emotional stressors like fear of loss or lack of support, resentment, obligation, environmental stressors like pollution, social media pressures and political unrest. It is important to find effective ways to cope with chronic stress by learning to activate the parasympathetic nervous system, which induces a state of calm, oversees rest and digestion and counterbalances the body's stress response.

Moreover, the uterus is negatively impacted by the stressful situation, potentially leading to an imbalance in the menstrual cycle. Chronic stress can wear down the body's natural defence mechanism and interfere with hormones,[121] adversely affecting overall health. It is essential to be vigilant of physical symptoms that may indicate stress-related issues.

True healing is a result of change—a shift in thoughts, beliefs and timely action. You hold the power to metamorphose through dedicated practice of daily yoga, pranayama and meditation, along with lifestyle changes. Yoga is a gentle, gradual, effective stress management tool that guides you to participate in the present moment. It redirects all your emotions from an anxious, fearful state to a joyful, creative one, by activating the parasympathetic nervous system.[122]

This greatly helps counter any negative thoughts and encourages gentle, rational, inner monologues in order to maintain a healthy balance between work and rest.

[121]Cassata, Cathy, 'Here's How Stress can Trigger a Hormonal Imbalance', *Healthline*, Healthline Media, 21 March 2019, https://www.healthline.com/health-news/hormone-imbalances-and-how-to-treat-them.

[122]Rice, Andrea, 'Yoga for Anxiety: 9 Poses to Try', *PsychCentral*, Healthline Media, 26 October 2021, https://psychcentral.com/anxiety/yoga-for-anxiety.

APPROACH TOWARDS YOGA

'Yoga is the journey of the self,
through the self, to the self.'

—THE BHAGAVAD GITA

Yoga is a versatile healing practice that can be tailored and adapted to suit every person's bodily needs, hormonal variations, gynaecological problems, mental health issues and age factors as each person is unique. It is not about how stiff the body is or how old you are. It is about how dedicated and disciplined you are towards your health.

The best way to learn yoga is through a trained teacher who can guide you to fine-tune your postures, suggest alternatives or additions to optimize your efforts and ensure that your breathing is in sync with each asana. The right teacher is the one who can motivate you to persevere and is compassionate enough to guide you through the entire session.

Yoga is the pursuit of spiritual insight and tranquillity. Various yogic disciplines or traditions, such as Hatha, Ashtanga, Iyengar, Vinyasa, Kundalini or Western yoga encompass distinct styles. Each school of yoga is different and may not be suitable for everyone. It is important to identify the most suited school for you and follow the practice diligently. This can ensure improved cognitive functions, better sleep, good appetite, more compassion and less negative self-talk and invariably good reproductive health.

HEALING THROUGH YOGA

- It boosts energy and ensures better sleep and a radiant glow.
- It is customizable, versatile and curative.

- Yogic postures increase mobility and protect you from potential injury.
- Twisting asanas aid digestion and metabolism, prevent constipation and bloating and increase blood circulation around the digestive tract.
- Yoga improves posture by strengthening and stretching the shoulders, chest, back and abdominals weakened by sedentary lifestyles.
- It reduces PMS symptoms by releasing happy hormones.
- It boosts confidence and increases capabilities by altering thoughts, patterns and intentions towards better health.
- It detoxifies the body through exhalation and sweat, eliminates tension and cleanses both body and mind.

These are just a few benefits of yoga.

HEALING THROUGH PRANAYAMA

'Breathing is the link between body and mind,
between spirit and matter,
between the conscious and the subconscious mind.'

—DAN BRULE

Breathing techniques can significantly build one's mental resilience when practised with patience and perseverance for about 5–10 minutes every day on an empty stomach.

The rhythm of breathing varies, affecting hormonal levels and leading to emotional and physical disturbances. Practising pranayama regularly by focusing on your lower abdomen helps regulate hormonal fluctuations. While some breathing patterns are designed to calm the inner self, others energize and invigorate the nervous system.

To achieve optimal health, it is crucial to grasp the

essence of breath, represented by the *nadis* or pathways of *ida* and *pingala* in Sanskrit. Ida is linked to the left nostril and symbolizes the Moon's (yin) energy of creativity and intuition while pingala is connected to the right nostril and embodies the Sun's (yang) energy of logic, vitality, and adventure. Both spiral along the spine and influence mental functions, easing the mind and soothing the body. Breath therapy is an inner practice that involves a series of deliberate breathing techniques, manipulating inhalations and exhalations through different breath retention patterns, leading to healing and rejuvenation.

Several forms of pranayama help to balance the ida and pingala energies. These powerful techniques can transform body dynamics. A few of them include:

- Kapalbhati (forceful exhalation)
- Nadi Shodhana (alternate nostril breathing)
- Surya Nadi (right-nostril breathing)
- Chandra Nadi (left-nostril breathing)
- Bhramari (bee breath)

All these breathing styles have individual curative benefits, and when practised under a trained yoga teacher, they can help address specific issues by cleansing all nadis (or chakras) to restore balance.

Nadi Shodhana pranayama, or alternate nostril breathing, is my go-to tool for calming my nerves and decluttering my mind. This simple breathing technique instantly balances the two hemispheres of the brain, clears blocked energy channels, and effectively handles daily stress. It is a blessing to have this powerful stress buster in our arsenal as it can be practised anywhere to soothe the mind—whether you find yourself stuck in bad traffic, facing a crucial decision or dealing with a challenging situation.

Combining yogic postures with proper breathing stimulates

the vagus nerve, which runs from the brain through the face, thorax and to the abdomen, activating the neurotransmitters of the gut.[123] This is the reason why you normally feel blissful and content after yoga. Remember that incorrect breathing patterns become the precursor to many ailments of the body and mind. Therefore, practising under the supervision of the right teacher is essential to recognize the art of pranayama. Breath is power, so use this weapon to your advantage by focusing on solutions

THE PHILOSOPHY OF YOGA

The science of yoga teaches that all matter in the cosmos is vibrant with life. It describes the Moon and the Sun as two omnipotent energies. A person is in an energized state when the breath is flowing out of the right (sun or pingala) nostril and in a passive state when the breath is flowing out of the left (moon or ida) nostril.

Yin/Moon Yoga

The practice of Yin, also restorative yoga, is a slower and cooler approach to physical activity, focusing on passive and seated postures. These *asanas* target the connective tissues in the hips, pelvis, lower spine and bones, bringing increased flexibility in reproductive organs and lower body parts while stimulating the production of oestrogen. By utilizing props like bolsters, blocks, chairs and bands, practitioners can hold these postures for extended periods, resulting in deep, transformative results.

These poses serve as a powerful tool to restore balance and tranquillity, tapping into the nurturing, creative and compassionate qualities associated with the feminine energy.

[123]Juliano-Villani, Gabrielle, 'Yogic Breathing: Types, Benefits, & Techniques,' *Choosing Therapy*, 12 April 2003, https://www.choosingtherapy.com/yogic-breathing/.

In today's fast-paced world, Yin yoga offers a peaceful escape, allowing the body to breathe in the present moment without resistance or the need to 'fix' anything.

Yang/Sun Yoga

These dynamic poses allow you to focus more on active, vigorous movements and are considered to be 'warming-up' *asanas*. Yang poses promote progesterone, increase blood flow and strengthen your stamina, improving stability and sustenance. They help maintain balance in the masculine side by working on the logical and analytical aspects of one's personality.

Women experience different levels of stress every day. To combat this, it is essential to strike the right balance of restorative and dynamic postures for different cycles. This can mitigate the negative effects of stress hormones. Embracing this deep wisdom is what steers you towards better well-being.

YOGA DURING MENSTRUATION

Practising *asanas* during menstruation has long been a subject of controversy, sparking numerous debates. However, after limiting my practice to restorative poses and experiencing numerous benefits, I feel compelled to assert that the primary objective of yoga poses is to support the body and the hormones and not work against it.

The menstrual phase is a downward process of elimination, dominated by downward wind energy. This wind, located in the large intestine, addresses the vital functions of menstruation and maintains all excretory processes. Understanding this science of downward energy flow needs a deep perception and is rightfully supported through silence and restive yoga poses, yoga nidra (yogic sleep) and gentle breathing techniques or pranayamas.

Menstruation is a powerful phase for women, offering a heightened level of sensitivity and awareness. However, different women deal with periods differently. Some treat their bodies with care and respect, allowing themselves to rest and recoup, while others push through discomfort and ignore the body's messages, risking potential harm.

During menstruation, the body is vulnerable to imbalances in the doshas, making it crucial to follow a healthy regimen for menstruation. Over-exerting the body through intense yoga, physical activities or sexual intercourse can create an internal conflict and disturb the delicate balance of hormones, leading to abnormal bleeding patterns, severe cramps and other psychosomatic or stress-related problems.

Thus, it is not recommended to practice inversions, twisting, bending and standing poses during menstruation as these types of yoga poses generate energy and can further disrupt the delicate balance of the body. Restorative yoga aims to address menstrual symptoms on a profound level along with nourishing food and adequate rest. The term 'rest' here implies not pushing yourself too hard but also not spending the entire day lying down on the couch. The daily schedules may demand otherwise but a deliberate slowing down and maintaining a certain degree of silence will naturally propel the body to be more productive in the days to come.

MY EXPERIENCE WITH YOGA

For decades, I've had the fortune of practising Iyengar Yoga under the guidance of renowned teacher H.S. Arun. This journey has been transformative, nurturing a profound bond with yoga that has revitalized both my body and mind. Arun's personalized approach to instruction, tailored to individual needs and concerns, has empowered me to confront my fears and embrace a therapeutic path to wellness. Through his guidance, I've gained a newfound perspective on life, cultivating abundance and inner resistance.

Even at the age of 61, yoga remains an integral part of my life, continually shaping my journey and enabling me to unlock my fullest potential.

Arun's book *Experiment & Experience on the Chair: The Yoga Way*, featuring a foreword by Guruji Dr B.K.S. Iyengar, is a great aid for women to work with props effortlessly. It offers insights into utilizing props effectively, catering to different body types (vata, pitta, kapha) and related moods, passions and sublimation of the ego. Beyond promoting holistic health, this book underscores the transformative power of yoga through props facilitating full extension, expansion and good circulation of the body—demonstrating that yoga transcends mere physical exercise.

YOGA FOR YOUR MENSTRUAL CYCLE

During menstruation, women often experience various physical symptoms, including nausea, dizziness, diarrhoea, breast tenderness, bloating, cramps, skin issues and abdominal or lower back pain. While prescription drugs and supplements can help regulate the hormones temporarily, yoga can provide complementary healing, addressing the root cause when practised mindfully under a qualified instructor. Yoga should not be viewed simply as a weight loss tool but as a holistic way to address menstrual problems. With regular practice, you will experience a sense of calm and develop the ability to handle adversity gracefully.

In this chapter, we will explore how yoga works on the body and mind during different menstrual phases, offering insights into tailored practices for each stage.

Phase 1: Menstrual Phase/Inner Winter (Days 1-5)

Releasing Mode
Place: Mind
Mood of the Phase: Night

Menstruation or the inner winter time of the month is governed by the wind element. With oestrogen levels at their lowest, the downward movement of wind element (*apana vayu*) is natural. Therefore, increasing the body's natural heightened awareness and sensitivity by maintaining silence is essential. This enables you to develop intuition towards comprehending clear and lucid messages from your body. Pay attention to these messages, as they hold the hidden clues guiding you to unravel the mysteries of life, gently nudging you to release emotions that may no longer serve you.

Engaging in physical extremes such as mindless scrolling, lying in bed all day or overwhelming oneself with too many activities can disturb the body's wind element, potentially manifesting as PMS symptoms later on. To combat this, individuals with sedentary lifestyles should make slight modifications by gently flexing the body at set intervals. Conversely, hyperactive individuals should make necessary changes to their hectic schedules by consciously delegating tasks or taking moments for relaxation.

To-dos during Wintertime

During menstruation, opting for restorative (yin) yoga poses can relieve pelvic and abdominal discomfort, mood swings and irritability. These poses bring peace and tranquillity to the mind and also strengthen the womb's health by enhancing the proper circulation of bodily fluids. Practising restorative poses during menstruation ensures a seamless transition to the next phase without complications.

Restorative/Yin Period Poses

1. Balasana or Child Pose
2. Chakravakasana or Cat Pose
3. Supta Baddha Konasana or Reclining Bound Angle Pose
4. Supta Virasana or Reclining Hero Pose
5. Paschimottanasana or Seated Forward Bend
6. Adho Mukha Virasana or Downward Facing Hero Pose
7. Setu Bandha Sarvangasana or Supported Bridge Pose
8. Janusirsasana or Head-to-Knee Pose
9. Baddha Konasana or Butterfly Pose
10. Upavistha Konasana or Seated Straddle Pose
11. Sukhasana or Easy Sitting Pose
12. Shavasana or Corpse Pose

- Unwinding with Shavasana can reduce symptoms of fatigue and anxiety. Mindful breathing, especially during shavasana and other supine postures, promotes the circulation of oxygen within the body, relaxes uterine muscles and soothes painful cramps.
- In addition to these restorative postures, leisurely walks without gadgets or slow, rhythmic dance movements can help keep endorphins high.
- Practicing Ujjayi pranayama and yoga nidra helps in balancing the energy channels of the body.
- Massaging castor oil around the navel, or using a hot compressor for the lower abdomen can relieve muscular pain.

Phase 2: Follicular Phase/Inner Spring (Days 6–11)

Rising Mode
Place: Eyes
Mood of the Phase: Morning

After the sabbatical wintertime, spring is governed by the water element with feelings of enthusiasm and vibrancy, symbolizing new beginnings. Oestrogen starts to rise along with FSH, which brings childlike enthusiasm and energy to match. The body and mind begin to feel revitalized after the bleeding phase.

To-dos during Springtime

Let this rising enthusiasm spread to the yoga mat after the downward and inward menstruation phase. Your practice can begin with the restive (yin) poses and gradually transition to dynamic and strengthening yang poses, concluding with shavasana. Utilize this super springtime by practising yoga poses to stimulate all the organs by incorporating backbends and reintroducing inversions to strengthen the core.

1. Bhujangasana or Cobra Pose
2. Dhanurasana or Bow Pose
3. Upavistha Konasana or Upright Wide-Angle Seated Forward Bend
4. Baddha Konasana
5. Natarajasana or Dancer Pose
6. Virabhadrasanas or six Warrior Pose variations
7. Yoga Inversion Poses
8. Yoga Backbends
9. Twisting Yoga Poses
10. Shavasana

- Inversion asanas target the thyroid and pituitary glands, strengthen muscles and regulate the body's metabolism.

- Pelvic poses can help to overcome fear and face new challenges in life.
- This is the time to practise new variations and poses. Explore difficult asanas without hesitation but under supervision.
- Increasing the intensity of other forms of physical activities such as swimming, biking or dancing releases kapha dosha, which helps to clear muddled thoughts.
- Lift, move, sprint and engage in lunges, side-planks, dips, burpees, crunches, upper and lower body pushes or strength training.
- Breathing techniques like Bhastrika and Kapalbhati can be therapeutic and balance your surging energy.

Phase 3: Ovulatory Phase/Inner Summer (Days 12–19)

Responding Mode
Place: Stomach
Mood of the Phase: Noon

The inner summertime of the menstrual cycle is governed by a fire element as women typically experience a rise in oestrogen. This results in increased energy and a feeling of vitality. This phase is the perfect time to be socially active, communicate with others, conceive new ideas and collaborate on projects. For those planning for motherhood, this phase is considered to be the best time for conception. Embrace the energy and strength of this phase by seizing opportunities and taking action towards your goals.

Hence, this is a good time to bring masculine (yang) energy to the fore by exploring postures under expert guidance.

Keep in mind that with the rise of adrenaline, it's important to soothe and manage your high-strung energy.

To-dos during Summertime

- Begin with more yang poses and complete them with a few yin (feminine) sequences.

    1. Sirsasana or Headstand Pose
    2. Ardha Chandrasana or Half Moon Pose and its Variations
    3. Urdhva Dhanurasana or Backbending Pose
    4. Surya Namaskara or Sun Salutation
    5. Balasana or Child Pose
    6. Bakasana or Crow Pose
    7. Astavakrasana or Eight-Angle Pose
    8. Shavasana

- Breathing exercises like Nadi Shodhana can help you to stay calm and become more focused without burning out.
- Balance the high-energy needs of this phase with cooling activities, such as the Sheetali pranayama, and incorporate endothermic food into your diet.
- Develop a healthy lifestyle strategy to optimize your body weight, adjusting food habits to support your hormones rather than solely focusing on weight loss. During this phase, the body utilizes fat as fuel, making it an opportune time to shed those extra kilos.
- Incorporate high-intensity interval training, strength training, brisk walks or faster movements of vinyasa yoga.
- Be mindful that any over-strenuous fitness regime may disrupt pitta dosha, leading to heavy flow and frequent clotting. Understand that the notion of adopting high metabolic rates for weight loss is a misconception.
- Prioritize good quality sleep and a nutritious diet, which can calm the heightened energy levels and provide relaxation for overworked organs.

Phase 4: Luteal Phase/Inner Monsoon/Fall (Days 20–26)

Reflective Mode
Place: Heart
Mood of the Phase: Dusk

As the hormones transition post-ovulation, the body is governed by the Earth element, readying for a fresh cycle. It is crucial to recognize the importance of balancing goals and aspirations with attention to personal well-being. Progesterone, a hormone that can fluctuate suddenly, can lead to unpredictable emotions and behaviour.

The inner monsoon phase is a moment for the body to treat its innermost feelings with gentleness. So embrace intentional pauses and foster grounding, creating an opportune time for introspection and reflection.

Permit yourself the space to unwind and reflect on the ideas, actions and accomplishments of the previous spring and summer phases without judgment.

To-dos during Monsoons/Fall

During the transition period, practice dynamic yang poses and gradually ease into restorative yin poses to mitigate the effects of PMS.

1. All standing asanas, such as Virabhadrasana, Trikonasana or Triangle Pose and Uttanasana or Standing Forward Bend
2. Kapotasana or Pigeon Pose
3. Inversions like Sarvangasana or Shoulder Stand, Sirsasana and Adho Mukha Svanasana or Downward Facing Dog Pose
4. Backbending, such as Bhujangasana, Dhanurasana,

Malasana or the Garland Pose, Deviasana or Goddess Pose and Baddha Konasana
5. Shavasana or Balasana

- Practise core-strengthening exercises, Pilates, strength training or outdoor exercises to release built-up energy.
- Pranayamas such as Kapalbhati and Anulom Vilom can calm your flustered mind.

YOGA—THE RIGHT WAY

'Yoga is not about touching your toes.
It is what you learn on the way down.'

—JIGAR GOR

Daily practice should give you the energy to get through your daily tasks. Do remember that menstrual bleeding varies in length, from person to person and from month to month, depending on the individual body type. Adopt and modify the right yogic sequences for your specific cycle to maximize your potential.

Practising three dimensions of yoga builds up resistance against discomforts and diseases. While embarking on the journey to good health often begins on the yoga mat, genuine transformation unfolds as you carry the wisdom gleaned from the mat through the diverse phases of your menstrual cycle. This profound insight empowers you to gracefully navigate the ebb and flow of discomforts and joys, lows and highs, fostering a newfound sense of acceptance free from resistance or judgment. It enables you to accept the present realities and welcome each cycle with optimism. This is the real essence of yoga.

THE BOTTOM LINE

Yoga is a discipline to be followed every day. So show up on the mat to organically heal your body and eliminate all the negative conditioning. Release the traumas of the past and the anxieties of the future to benefit from the present moment. This is the real yoga that you need to aim for. Along with practising asanas, pranayama and meditation to strengthen your womb energy, get the right vitamins, green up your diet, maintain healthy habits and align your lifestyle with your menstrual cycle.

NIMMI'S MANTRA

Yoga teaches the art of breathing through challenges and finding calm in the storm.

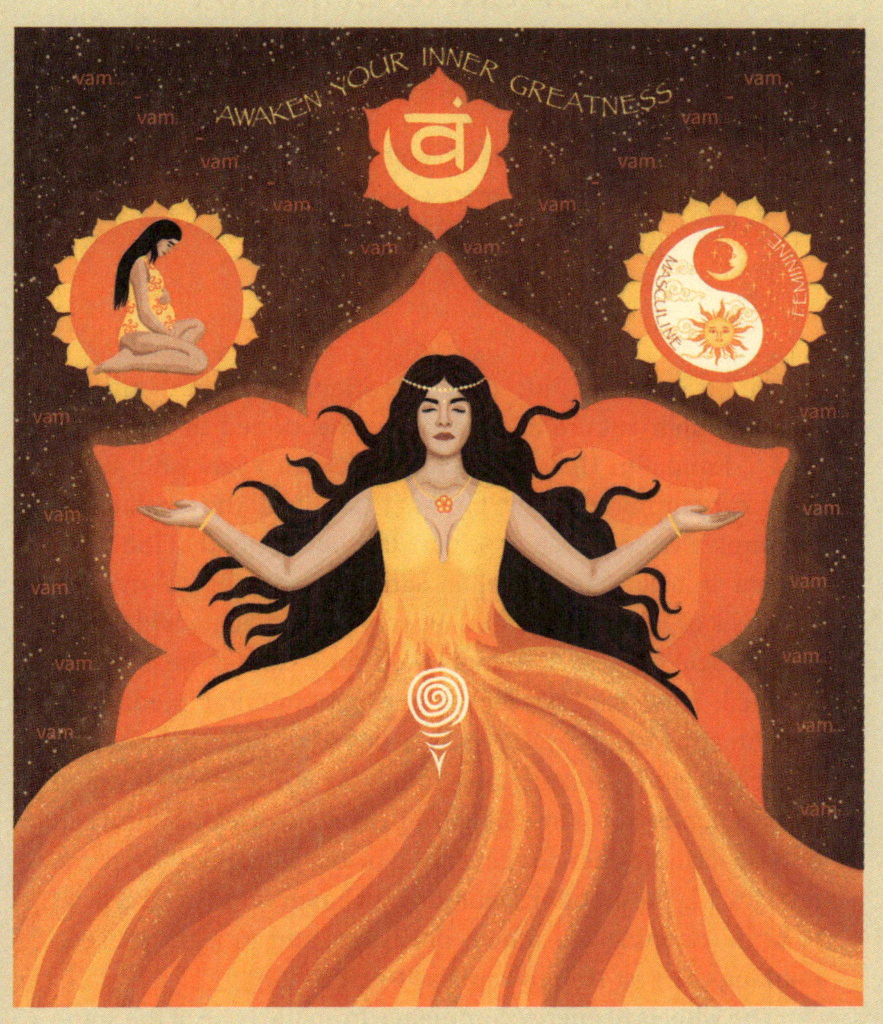
AWAKEN YOUR INNER GREATNESS
vam
MASCULINE
FEMININE

14

THE SACRAL CHAKRA

'Energy speaks louder than words.
Change your energy, change your life.'

—ANONYMOUS

The concept of chakras originates from ancient Indian culture and has been mentioned in the Yoga-Kundalini Upanishad. It was Indian yogis who, using their extraordinary yogic powers, identified the chakras as a complex energy system within the human body. The term 'chakra' translates to 'wheel' in Sanskrit and refers to invisible channels of life force (pranic) energy that circulate within us.

Though chakras are intangible and cannot be seen or touched, they can be sensed through mindful meditation and breathwork. They serve as a powerful link between the conscious and subconscious mind. As the conscious mind comprehends words and language, the subconscious mind can only absorb the energies generated by our thoughts. Therefore, recognizing the emotions vibrating within the chakras is crucial to understanding our mood, behaviour and thought process, marking the first step towards self-realization.

The wheels of energy commence from the base of the spine and extend to the crown of the head, enabling the flow of life force (*prana*) throughout the body. The flow of chakra becomes a reflection of our emotional and physical well-being. The Seven

Chakras, which are present within every human body, are ever-changing and influence every decision we make. Although they are dynamic and fluctuating, they have the power to assist you in transforming your inner self.

THE SEVEN CHAKRAS

Each of the seven major chakras is represented by a specific number of lotus petals. They are aligned from the lowest to the highest based on their positioning in the body, corresponding to the major gland with which each chakra is associated. In modern times, Western and Eastern cultures recognize this as a form of metaphysics and acknowledge its proximity with the endocrine system and the nervous system along with their associated organs.[124]

Understanding the seven major chakras can unlock your hidden potential and help you attain self-realization. By learning to identify the energetic pattern of each chakra, you can determine whether they are vibrating at higher or lower frequency levels—this, in turn, can assist you in decoding your emotions and behaviour. Balancing these chakras can improve our mental and menstrual well-being.

Location of seven major chakras:

- Muladhara (or the Root Chakra) is located at the base of the spinal cord, between the anus and the genitals, and is associated with the adrenal gland.
- Svadhisthana (or the Sacral/Pelvic Chakra) is located in the lower abdomen two inches below the navel and is related to

[124]Leland, Kurt, 'The Rainbow Body: How the Western Chakra System Came to Be', *The Theosophical Society in America*, https://www.theosophical.org/publications/quest-magazine/the-rainbow-body-how-the-western-chakra-system-came-to-be.

the ovarian gland in females and testicular glands in males.

- Manipura (or the Naval Chakra) is found two inches above the navel in the stomach area and is connected to the pancreas.
- Anahata (or the Heart Chakra) is located in the heart region and is linked with the thymus.
- Vishuddhi (or the Throat Chakra) is located at the base of the throat and corresponds to the thyroid gland.
- Ajna (or the Third-eye Chakra) is situated between the eyebrows and connected to the pituitary gland.
- Sahasrara (or the Crown Chakra) is located at the crown of the head and is connected to the pineal gland.

Each chakra possesses its own vibrational frequency, depicted through specific sounds, mantras, colours, numbers and names. They are strategically positioned along the length of the spine to govern specific functions in the body. Mastering the art of 'balancing chakras' can create intrinsic harmony and maintain relationships with those around us.

As a dedicated chakra therapist, the subtle energy system has provided me with profound insight and has enabled me to make conscious choices, allowing me to channel my effort and resources towards unlocking my full potential.

This has significantly helped me remain centred and grounded, avoiding reactive or ego-driven actions that could have led to wasted efforts. I have gained the ability to experience both pain and pleasure with composure, and have strived to guide others through the process of clearing imbalanced energies.

EXPLORING THE SACRAL CHAKRA

Having understood the basics of chakras, let us traverse the Svadhisthana/Sacral Chakra because of its correlation with the womb. Svadhisthana, which means the dwelling place of the self, explores the expansion of creativity, desires and sexuality. This enables us to enjoy all relationships and social experiences with grace and enthusiasm. It is an essential chakra for women to maintain stability and balance due to its powerful influence on reproductive health.

Symbols and Positions

- Image: 'The six-petal lotus', with each petal representing a negative trait of human nature (wrath, hate, jealousy, cruelty, lust and pride) to overcome.
- Position: Located three inches below the navel (pelvic area), where the coccyx and the sacrum meet.
- Colour: Orange, symbolizing activity, energy, joy and hope
- Mantra: Vam
- Element: Water, signifying soft and yielding
- Animal: Crocodile, representing lethargy
- Symbol: Half Moon, indicating feelings, tides, female cycle
- Divinity: Brahma (creator, consciousness) and Saraswati (knowledge, intellect, discrimination)
- Feature: Rasa, meaning fluidity
- Organs: The lower abdomen (reproductive organs), large intestine, lymphatic system, spleen and the appendix
- Heal: Address self-guilt, shame, anger
- Yantra: Crescent Moon
- Mind: Unconscious
- Centre: A focal point for passion, pleasure and creativity
- The seat of Shiva and Shakti, symbolizing the union of masculine and feminine energies.

THE SPIRITUAL CONNECTION

'I am radiant, beautiful, creative and strong; and I enjoy a healthy and passionate life.'

—ANONYMOUS

The womb embodies the entirety of our soul's journey and karmas across all lifetimes, acting as a repository, storing the imprints of every past experience, including each sexual encounter, regardless of their nature. This sacred space is influenced by the experiences of childbirth and abortion, carrying within it inherited ancestral patterns. These patterns weave into the fabric of one's emotional, physical and spiritual realms, significantly influencing the dynamics of relationships.[125]

It is vital for women to recognize that healthy menstruation signifies a balanced Svadhisthana Chakra spiritually connected to the uterus (womb) and its associated hormones. The energy of Svadhisthana fluctuates with every menstrual cycle; for example, our inner passion peaks during ovulation (inner summer) but cannot be sustained during the luteal phase (inner monsoon/fall). While these emotional and behavioural changes are nature-ordained, making conscious adjustments to our daily routine and adopting new perspectives can help balance this chakra and promote a healthy life. The more we lay down our defences to relax, the more our bodies can naturally heal and rebalance. This wisdom empowers women to gain the clarity and mental resilience required to manoeuvre in life.

[125] de la Agua, Angela, 'Womb Chakra,' *Sacred Motherhood Blueprint*, 2 April 2020, https://www.sacredmotherhoodblueprint.com/musings/2020/4/1/awakening-to-your-holy-womb-chakra.

The essence of the Womb Chakra is to maintain the balance between both feminine and masculine energy. In balancing these binaries, it highlights qualities such as passion, creativity, longing, nurturing, intuition, vibrancy, fluidity, sensuality, receptivity, adaptability, self-assurance and expressiveness, all of which are nurtured through the Sacral Chakra.

IDENTIFYING THE IMBALANCE

As Svadhisthana is the creative centre of the body, any imbalance that disrupts the natural flow of creativity can lead to negative emotions such as anger, hatred, jealousy, stubbornness, excessive dependency and emotional instability.

Blockage in the Womb Chakra can create an urge to indulge in worldly pleasures, fantasies and sexual obsessions. It may also lead to contradicting behavioural traits such as experiencing sexual frigidity, feelings of detachment or an emotionally explosive, irritable and manipulative personality. Women not in tune with this chakra can become aggressive and insecure and constantly seek validation from others. Inner child issues might also crop up unexpectedly, creating internal turmoil and magnifying feelings of shame and guilt.

An underactive chakra leads to emotional blockages within the body, giving rise to fear, anxiety, sadness and self-doubt, which consecutively create addictions to mood enhancers like caffeine, tea, alcohol, drugs or sweets. If not addressed timely, these unhealthy patterns can eventually affect menstrual and mental health with multiple reproductive issues such as infertility, ovarian cysts, endometriosis, urinary tract infection and depression.

Disturbances in the functioning of one chakra can unsettle other chakras, as they are interdependent and operate as a single entity. Over time, they can cause disruptions in related organs and lead to various physical ailments and diseases. The symptoms may look extensive and worrisome, but we need to remember that chakras are fluid and fluctuating, so any imbalance can be treated by early intervention.

BALANCING THE SACRAL CHAKRA

To heal and balance the Sacral Chakra, different components like colours, nutrition, water, yoga, meditation, etc., can be utilized.

Below are simple yet effective techniques to stay connected with this creative feminine hub and develop a healthier personal relationship with different phases of the menstrual cycle.

1. *Healing through Yoni Mudra*

Yoni Mudra is a symbolic representation of the vulva or womb (uterus) and the word 'mudra' means hand position. In Hinduism, the yoni mudra is dedicated to Goddess Kali—a symbol of strength and mystery. Practising Yoni Mudra meditation helps you to connect with your innate creative, female energy and detach yourself from the chaos of the outer world. Regular practice can aid in overcoming reproductive health issues and hormonal imbalances and also improve fertility.

This mudra can be performed at any time of the day. Sit in a comfortable posture with your spine straight either in Padmasana (Lotus) or Sukhasana (Cross-legged posture), as these postures create a beautiful aura by making the energy move in a circle around you. The yoni mudra is a powerful practice to calm the mind. Place your index fingers and thumb in a triangle form and interlock the rest of your fingers right below the navel. With your eyes closed, bring your focus on the Womb Chakra. Visualize the life force spreading its warm, orange light throughout the entire pelvic region. Feel the Womb Chakra vibrating with feminine power, expanding your consciousness to higher dimensions with every deep breath you inhale.

2. *Healing through Mantra*

The Sacral Chakra vibrates with the sound Vam (pronounced v-uh-m), which was created thousands of years ago. This sound enables the flow of cosmic energies to cleanse past traumas and karma. Sages from the Vedic era understood how repetitions of mantras can influence the brain. Harnessing this unique power, they crafted powerful vibrations through Beej (meaning seed) mantras, which cleared blocked emotions and activated all the chakras.

Before chanting these mantras, seat yourself comfortably away from the noise. Chant the Vam mantra loudly with deep inhalation and exhalation by focusing your attention on your lower pelvis. Use beads (*malas*) to keep count of your chants and practice the ritual consistently. Mantras are typically chanted in multiples of 9 (e.g., 9, 18, 27, ..., 108 or 1,111 times and more) and gradually increase the count over time. Regular practice of this mantra can energize the Sacral Chakra and clear blocked emotions.

3. *Healing through Sound/Music*

'There is nothing in the world
so much like prayer as music is.'

—WILLIAM SHAKESPEARE

Certain sound frequencies are powerful enough to increase the vibrations of the womb and bring positive life changes.[126]

[126]'Reclaim Your Womb: Healing Through RRT and Reiki Sound Therapy,' *Glisten with Jac,* 18 November 2023, https://www.glistenwithjac.com/blog/reclaim-your-womb-healing-through-rrt-and-reiki-sound-therapy.

Blocked emotions can be cleared by listening to the 417 Hz frequency as it is associated with Sacral Chakra healing.[127]

Listening to binaural beats in a tranquil environment or while performing mundane tasks can bolster the potency of specific brain waves. Any sound that resonates within your soul can be played in the background during daily activities, effectively increasing the energy vibrations of the womb.

Repetitive exposure to a rhythmic sound can induce a trance-like state. This phenomenon has been observed across various cultures that use unique sound therapies to activate the feminine chakras. These therapeutic methods include invigorating sounds, chanting mantras, Tibetan singing bowls, Sufi melodies, and drumming therapy, as they help in healing the subconscious mind.

In my journey of self-discovery, listening to healing sounds, mantras and diverse music genres has greatly facilitated my internal healing and amplified the sensitivity of my creative centre. Over the years, I've curated and delved into personal playlists featuring both Eastern and Western artists, effectively dissolving emotional blockages. Consequently, this subtle shift has enhanced my creative feminine power and enabled me to pursue my interests with unwavering fervour.

Major illnesses such as depression, stress, autoimmune diseases, insomnia and reproductive or gut issues signify that the Sacral Chakra is vibrating at a lower frequency. Practising sound healing daily, using specific audio tones, can repair damaged tissues and cells within the body and help overcome traumatic experiences, broken relationships and depression. The gradual rise in energy can help you to vibrate at higher frequencies.

---

[127]Smith, Clare, 'What Are Chakra Frequencies? (Ultimate Guide)', *Chakra Practice*, https://chakrapractice.com/what-are-chakra-frequencies-ultimate-guide/.

Listening to 'Om' (pronounced aum) mantras, vibrating music or specific sound frequencies, especially during dawn and dusk, are powerful and rejuvenating meditative practices. The right frequency can instantly make you feel calmer and more positive.

4. *Healing through Affirmations*

'An affirmation opens the door.
It's a beginning point on the path to change.'

—LOUISE HAY

Verbal or written affirmations can resonate deeply within the Womb Chakra, alleviating negative energy blockages. Practice these positive affirmations regularly along with other mindful practices to bring about transformation:

- I am a unique, creative and powerful being.
- I lead a life full of passion and purpose.
- I fully embrace and celebrate my sexuality.
- I am free to flow and move with ease.
- I am comfortable and confident in my physical body.
- I am emotionally balanced and grounded.

To further manifest the change you desire, create your own affirmations and repeat them consistently for at least 21 days with unwavering faith. Witness the powerful and positive shifts that occur within your energy centre.

5. *Healing through Colour*

'Colour is a power
which directly influences the soul.'

—WASSILY KANDINSKY

Mother Nature thrives in rich, vibrant colours and glowing hues. Colours have a psychological effect on humans by awakening our innermost feelings; when colour transmits from the retina to the brain, they release hormones that affect emotions, clarity and energy.[128]

The Sacral Chakra is governed by the vibrant orange—a colour that makes you feel energized and enthusiastic without fear or self-doubt. Orange is the colour of purity and indicates positive qualities such as joy, faith and self-confidence.

Activate your sensuality, growth and pleasure by harnessing the energy of the vibrant orange colour through your Sacral Chakra. Mindfully choose orange-hued clothing, decor and nourishment, including spices, fruits, vegetables, vibrant flowers or an orange colour bottle to drink water from to invigorate your chakra's power and boost positive emotions.

6. *Healing through Nature*

'I have a therapist, and her name is Nature.'

—ANONYMOUS

Deepen your connection with Svadhisthana Chakra by engaging with nature, especially spending time around water bodies such as ponds, streams, lakes or oceans. The tranquil sounds of water element can ease tension and foster positive emotions, revitalizing your chakra and releasing blocked energies.

Even if access to natural water bodies is not possible, taking a warm or cold shower with Epsom or sea salts can be an equally potent alternative to release negative thoughts and rigid attitudes stored subconsciously. By tapping into your womb/

[128]Koltuska-Haskin, Barbara, 'How Colors Affect Brain Functioning,' *Psychology Today*, 29 January 2023, https://www.psychologytoday.com/us/blog/how-my-brain-works/202301/how-colors-affect-brain-functioning.

feminine energy, you can effectively heal emotional wounds and amplify your creative potential. This can also strengthen your relationship with yourself and others.

7. Healing through Forgiveness and Gratitude

'Every woman who heals herself
helps heal all the women
who came before her,
and all those who will come after her.'

—CHRISTIANE NORTHRUP

Our ancestors honoured Nature's signals and messages by respecting every outcome without the pursuit of perfect solutions. Healing the womb by directing energy towards the Sacral Chakra was one such ritual of expressing gratitude for being born a woman. Our predecessors addressed all menstrual discomforts through rituals during the new moon and full moon days.

To heal the Womb Chakra is to address unresolved inner child issues and the ancestral karmas that may be blocking growth. Begin by forgiving your parents and gradually extend forgiveness to the rest of your family, including extended relatives, your spouse and friends. This process of forgiveness and acceptance can liberate your inner child by replacing negative thoughts with positive ones. Ultimately, this helps you become a responsible adult who takes action to release past ancestral karmas by first forgiving yourself and then others, enabling you to foster healthy relationships and attract greater prospects. This significantly helps future generations experience freedom from unresolved traumas and unhealthy attachments stored in this energy centre.

Here is a simple and effective ritual to follow whenever life feels disheartening. Begin by sitting on a chair or a mat with your back against the wall to maintain a straight posture. Then close your eyes, take slow breaths and place both hands on your lower belly. Inhale consciously, allowing your belly to expand, and open your heart to embrace life's gifts, inviting an attitude of gratitude for all things; with each deep exhalation, let go of pain, unease and stagnation, simultaneously seeking forgiveness and healing. Practice this ritual daily for 10–15 minutes and increase the duration as needed.

8. *Healing through Essential Oils*

'One drop at a time and you will get there;
It's all about nourishing your senses.'

—ANONYMOUS

Essential oils have a centuries-old history of treating ailments due to their instant relieving and relaxing effects. These oils are potent, with highly individual properties, and must be used in diluted forms to be effective. Concentrated essential oils should be mixed with carrier oils (vegetable/nut oil) or water in the diffuser device before use. Oils like vanilla, lemon, orange, ginger, sage, citrus, rose, jasmine, bergamot, geranium, ylang-ylang, patchouli and sandalwood are often used to heal the sensual Sacral Chakra. They can be used during prayers, meditations or even in baths, as they soothe nerves and relax muscles.

9. *Healing through Crystals and Stones*

'You know the world is a magical place
when Mother Earth grows her own jewellery.'

—ANONYMOUS

Crystals are known as nature's gift to augment healing, offering an alternative medicinal technique that taps into natural healing energy. Crystals are used to balance chakras that are either overactive or underactive, acting as conduits for healing by enabling positive energy to flow into the body. They are used along with orthodox medicine or other complementary therapies.

Scientific studies state that crystal structures and stones can collect, store and emit electromagnetic energy. Since these crystals are natural and extracted from the Earth, they can harness the energies of the Sun, Moon and oceans. Stones such as amber, citrine, moonstone, tiger's eye, carnelian and orange calcite are particularly effective in elevating the vibrations of the Sacral Chakra. To benefit from their energy, place them strategically around your home, carry them in a bag or pocket or wear them as jewellery.

Given that crystals absorb surrounding energies, they require thorough cleansing, which can be achieved by running them under water, exposing them to natural sunlight or energizing them with mantras or prayers.

10. *Healing with Herbs and Spices*

'The art of healing comes from nature, not from the physician. Therefore, the physician must start from nature, with an open mind.'

—PARACELSUS

Believe in the magical power of herbs and spices for their healing and medicinal properties. A simple herbal tea or concoction made from coriander, turmeric, ginger and fennel can promote relaxation by soothing digestive and abdominal muscles and improve gut health.

11. *Healing through Yoga*

'Yoga is for everyone.
No one is too old or too stiff, too fat or thin or tired.'

—B.K.S. IYENGAR

Every woman is unique and so is her womb. Here are some womb-centric yoga asanas that focus on uterine health and help maintain a healthy womb to support its vitality:

- Upavistha Konasana or Upright Wide-Angle Seated Forward Bend
- Baddha Konasana or Butterfly Pose
- Anjaneyasana or Low-lunge Pose
- Malasana or Garland Pose
- Utkata Konasana or Goddess Pose
- Virasana or Hero Pose

Practising these slow and rhythmic feminine poses can enhance the feminine energy and intimacy of this creative centre.

12. *Healing through Art and Creativity*

'The one you are looking for is you.'

—OSHO

Express yourself creatively and let it flow freely. Colour the canvas, dance to your favourite tunes, experiment with new recipes, compose music, spend time with kids or write in a journal. Dive into all art forms and rekindle forgotten childhood passions, as they can bring a sense of fulfilment and harmony, enhancing the energy flow to your Womb Chakra.[129]

[129]Wauters, Ambika, *Book of Chakras: Discover the Hidden Forces Within You*, Barron's Educational Series Inc., Hauppauge, NY, 18 April 2002.

THE BOTTOM LINE

An aligned chakra kindles every cell in the body, making thoughts and actions flexible and adaptable to the present time and space. It enables you to celebrate your strengths and accept your weaknesses with grace. Implement subtle yet necessary changes in your daily routine that will have a positive effect on your menstrual health. Activate your Womb Chakra to form an intrinsic bond with it and fulfil your life's purpose.

NIMMI'S MANTRA

Discipline and devotion are key to recognizing your true desires. Begin by loving all dimensions of yourself. Forgive yourself for past mistakes and acknowledge the joy and blessings around you. Consciously connect with your Womb Chakra to come home to yourself.

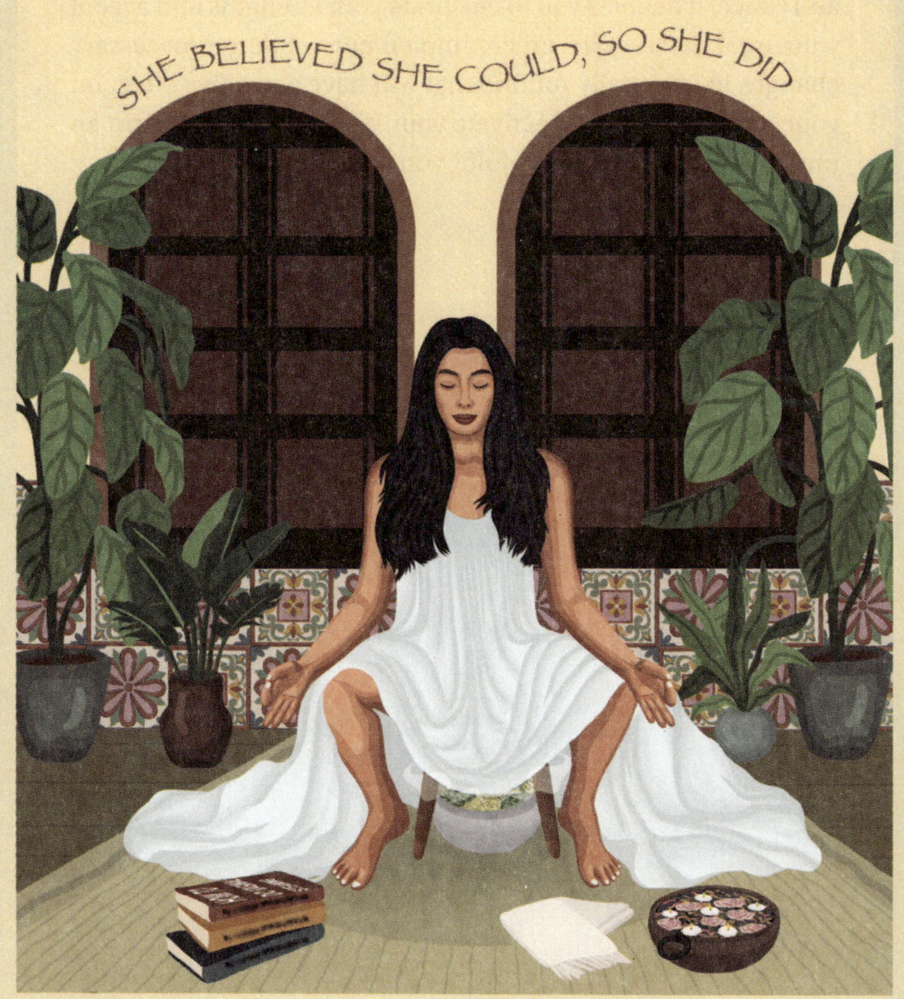
SHE BELIEVED SHE COULD, SO SHE DID

15

THE YONI RITUAL

'My yoni is a lush garden that encompasses a waterfall and when my desire is met, it overflows.'

—ANONYMOUS

Throughout history, rituals have been known to align with prevailing societal values. One such practice is yoni (or vaginal) steaming, which was widely popular among indigenous women in Asia and Africa.[130] This ritual was considered sacred and served to connect women with the strength and power of their wombs, enhancing creativity, fertility, sexual pleasure and overall wellness while mitigating menstrual symptoms.

The term 'yoni' is derived from Sanskrit and signifies the female genitalia, specifically the vulva. It symbolizes the worship of Goddess Shakti, embodying the essence of life and creativity. This concept holds deep reverence in both Hinduism and Buddhism. Yoni steaming is an important ceremony, retaining its relevance in contemporary times and carrying profound significance in the lives of many women.

[130]'Empowerment and Connection: Exploring the Cultural Roots of Yoni Steaming,' *Onyeka Tefari Wellness & Spa,* https://onyekatefari.com/empowerment-and-connection-exploring-the-cultural-roots-of-yoni-steaming/.

BENEFITS OF VAGINAL STEAMING

In our highly competitive and male-dominated world, rituals serve as crucial anchors to reconnect with our inner feminine essence. These mood-elevating practices assist women in untangling muddled-up thoughts and tapping into their innate goddess power.

Throughout a woman's life, her vagina endures significant pressures from menstruation, sexual intercourse, hormonal variations, childbirth and menopause. Over time, the Sacral or Womb Chakra absorbs a lot of emotions, leading to blocked energies. Yoni/vaginal rituals offer a conscious release of these suppressed emotions, enabling women to break free from inner turmoil and wounded inner child issues, resulting in a deeply cleansing and rejuvenating experience.

Today, vaginal steaming has been revived by modern society due to its revitalizing and energizing properties. It redirects women to improve their menstrual health by reconnecting to their source. Incorporating this practice into your self-care regimen can provide you with a profound sense of relaxation, emotional balance and self-awareness.

Yoni/vaginal steaming as a self-care ritual using natural herbs offers a multitude of benefits. It reconnects individuals with their womb energy, increases blood circulation to the vaginal area, regulates the menstrual cycle, eases period cramps, boosts libido, increases fertility, reduces vaginal dryness, promotes restful sleep and enables the release of toxic emotions such as stress, stubbornness and stagnation.[131]

Indeed, many women value this holistic approach to self-care, acknowledging it as a means of cultivating a magnetic

[131]'How to Yoni Steam at Home: Best Herbs, Benefits & DIY Setup', *Naema Pierce*, 7 June 2023, https://www.naemapierce.com/articles/how-to-yoni-steam-at-home-guide.

inner environment to absorb and radiate energies, and organically fostering overall growth and healing.

YONI INFUSION

Yoni infusion can bring about immense changes in overall wellness if practised regularly. It is an indigenous ritual that helps women to enjoy harmonious menstrual cycles.[132]

1. As a first step, choose a good quality yoni stool.
2. Choose natural and organic herbs as they are more effective and safer on your skin.
3. As prior preparation, soak one cup of dry herbs such as basil, rosemary and chamomile in a pot of steaming hot water (1–2 litres) for a couple of minutes. Avoid using essential oils or fragrances.
4. Set the yoni stool in a cosy room and place the herb-steeped pot underneath it.
5. Ensure the steam is not too hot and you feel comfortable with the temperature. Sit/squat comfortably without any undergarments to enable the healing vapours to penetrate.
6. A thick blanket or gown wrapped around the waist can prevent the steam from escaping as it rises, allowing the herbs to penetrate the vaginal area.
7. This therapeutic ritual works well when combined with soothing background music to keep the mind calm and serene.
8. Mute external disturbances to focus internally on your intimate area. Allow yourself an undistracted 20–30

[132]'Yoni Steaming: The Ancient Self-Care Practice for Loving Your Vagina,' *Paavani Ayurveda*, 13 May 2022, https://paavaniayurveda.com/blogs/the-ayurvedic-lifestyle/yoni-steaming-the-ancient-self-care-practice-for-loving-your-vagina.

minutes for this revitalizing infusion to work its magic.

9. Lie down for at least a few minutes after the ritual to feel the energy from the intimate area transmitting itself throughout the body.
10. Invest your time in creating a consistent yoni ritual and start to understand what it feels like to connect with your powerful centre.
11. Most importantly, practise using the right words to acknowledge and appreciate your yoni.

LOVE YOUR YONI

Embrace self-love and healing through the practice of affirmations while nurturing your yoni. Yoni steaming is a powerful tool that aligns the three pillars of holistic health—mind, body and soul. As you begin your yoni healing journey, it is crucial to set meaningful and impactful intentions.

Incorporate these empowering yoni affirmations into your practice:

- My yoni is a sacred centre of divine femininity.
- My yoni is sensual and sexual.
- My yoni is a source of creativity and joy.
- My yoni is a place of endless possibilities.
- My yoni is supportive and empathetic.

Channelling your energy into these affirmations offers a powerful means to liberate yourself from the lingering effects of negative self-talk, body shaming, self-hate, jealousy, anger and sadness. This transformative journey holds the potential to greatly uplift both your menstrual and mental well-being. Through this process, you can foster a profound connection with your body, strengthen relationships with loved ones and cultivate a deeper understanding and appreciation for yourself.

HERBAL REMEDIES

'A woman should always feel like spring;
scented and in a perpetual state of blossom.'

—ANONYMOUS

Yoni steaming is a powerful technique for enhancing optimal menstrual and reproductive health, providing an array of benefits such as alleviating vaginal yeast infections, enhancing sexual desire and toning vaginal muscles.[133] This ancient practice is often likened to a sauna for the vagina, as it relieves tensions in and around the pelvic region.

To initiate a successful yoni steaming regimen, it is essential to source natural and organic herbs that are either fresh or dried. A personalized blend can be crafted or pre-made herbal blends can be acquired based on individual needs. A range of herbs such as basil, ginger, mint, red rose, marigold, rosemary, lavender, sagebrush and oak bark are often combined for multiple benefits. These herbal blends can alleviate pain or discomfort associated with menstruation and directly nourish the reproductive area to hydrate, cleanse, purify and invigorate.

For instance, red rose petals are believed to possess uplifting and soothing effects on the uterus, motherwort has been observed to promote blood circulation and alleviate pain, chamomile is considered useful in treating amenorrhea (absent periods) while calendula is highly effective in rejuvenating womb energy.

[133]Vilma, '23 Benefits of Yoni Steam with Vaginal Risk, Safe Use', *Hei Mom*, 1 February 2023, https://heimom.com/yoni-steam/.

THE RIGHT TIME

Yoni steaming is best practised before and after menstruation. It is also an excellent post-delivery treatment.[134] However, women with intrauterine devices (IUDs), infection, sensitive skin or those pregnant or menstruating should consult a doctor before practising yoni steaming. The multiple positive effects are reflected in normalizing hormonal imbalances and eliminating menstrual discomfort. Regular practice helps to improve low moods and fosters mental clarity.

'May your mind, heart, and yoni align
to create a sensual and satisfying experience.'

—ANONYMOUS

THE BOTTOM LINE

The Yoni ritual is an essential step towards enhancing the intuitive mind. Such rituals are great ways to rekindle a woman's proximity to her sexuality. Let the healing journey enhance creativity, intimacy and sensual and orgasmic experiences not just within yourself but also between partners. Let us acknowledge and benefit from the virtue of our safe, indigenous rituals.

NIMMI'S MANTRA

Healing can happen on different levels. Allow yourself to be open and receptive to receive all its goodness by honouring your sacred sexuality.

[134] Meekins, Jamie, 'Yoni Steaming for Postpartum Recovery,' *Center for Sacred Window Studies*, https://sacredwindowstudies.com/2020/04/29/yoni-steaming-for-postpartum-recovery/.

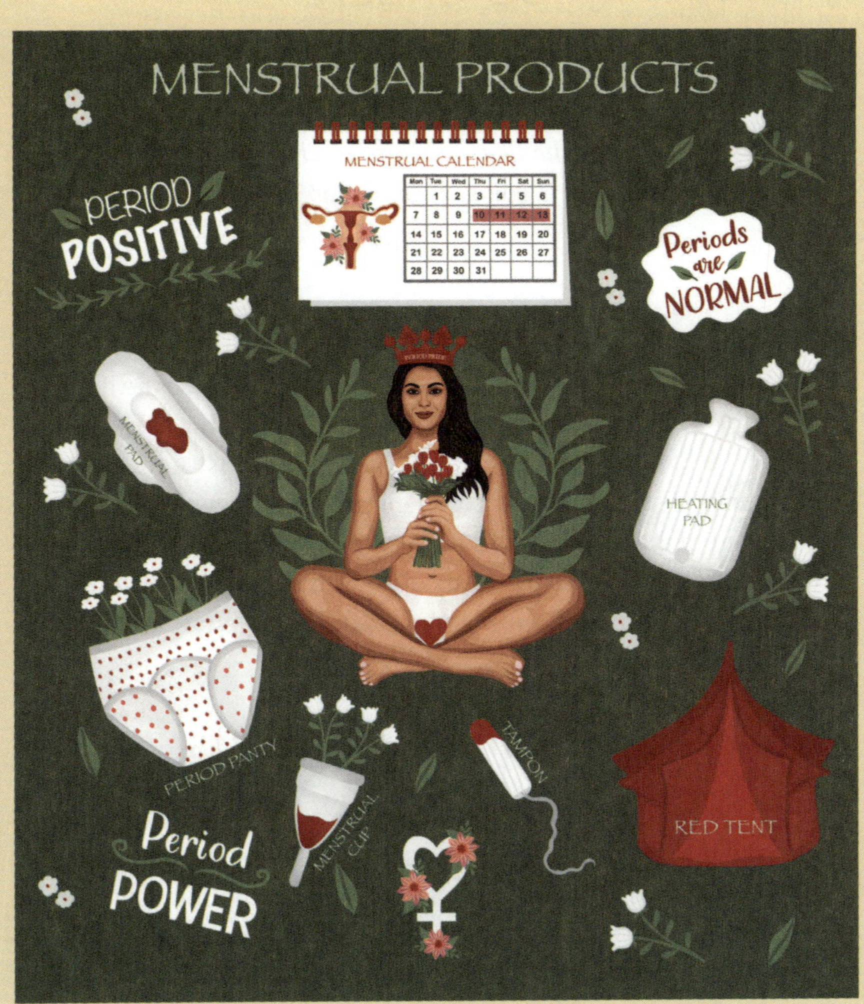
MENSTRUAL PRODUCTS
MENSTRUAL CALENDAR
Mon Tue Wed Thu Fri Sat Sun
1 2 3 4 5 6
7 8 9 10 11 12 13
14 15 16 17 18 19 20
21 22 23 24 25 26 27
28 29 30 31
PERIOD POSITIVE
Periods are NORMAL
MENSTRUAL PAD
HEATING PAD
PERIOD PANTY
TAMPON
RED TENT
MENSTRUAL CUP
Period POWER

16

GO GREEN

'Unless someone like you cares a whole awful lot, nothing is going to get better. It's not.'

—DR SEUSS

Women have navigated menstruation since the dawn of time, employing various methods for menstrual management. The Museum of Menstruation and Women's Health unveils a bygone era where women were confined to their homes and used cloth material or repurposed clothing as makeshift pads to absorb the blood, illustrating women's resilience, resourcefulness and innovation in period management.

SINGLE-USE MENSTRUAL PRODUCTS

In today's world, it is crucial for women to have access to safe, sustainable menstrual products such as reusable cloth pads and menstrual cups. While single-use pads and tampons may offer convenience for busy working women, this concept of presumed comfort has come with many added harmful materials that contain bleaches, additives, plastics, rayon and other chemicals, posing long-term risks to women and the environment.

The progressive world led us to believe that one-time (disposable) pads were the solution for 'free' time. Many of us enjoy the hygienic convenience of these disposable products. However, they are not eco-friendly, as the plastics in disposable pads end up in landfills and take hundreds of years to disintegrate. While we may have learned to cope with the aches and pains of menstruation that come with our monthly cycle, our planet is suffering from destruction caused by single-use plastic clogging up the oceans every year.

We are progressing exponentially as a society and have come a long way from using makeshift menstrual pads. However, not all menstrual products are created equal. We should be aware of certain toxic materials used in different products, which can pose potential health hazards to reproductive health in the long run.

It is time to wake up to the fact that menstrual experiences can be made pleasant and comfortable with biodegradable, compostable and organic options. Considering the importance of menstrual awareness, this chapter aims to enlighten women on the prevalent products, making it convenient for all women to personalize their 'period' moments.

PERSONALIZED PRODUCTS

Can we really make an impact on the planet by individually practising a zero-waste period?

As our experience with our periods has evolved, so have our menstrual products. In the past, women prioritized motherhood. However, priorities have now shifted and so have our bodies. On average, a woman menstruates for 3–7 days every month for almost 30 years of her life, totalling more than 400 periods in her lifetime; so inarguably, women must establish a closer bond with their womb and base their choice of menstrual products responsibly.

Over the years, menstrual products have also journeyed

from rags to hygienic cotton, disposable pads, leak-proof, eco-friendly and finally sustainable alternatives. There has been an emergence of organic, unbleached cotton tampons that are free from pesticides and genetically modified organisms. These developments have resulted in a plethora of options and have taken the feminine hygiene industry by storm. Today, there are menstrual products of various shapes and sizes that are less wasteful and more environmentally friendly. It is essential to consider the eco-friendliness of these products while choosing from the many options available, ensuring they are safe for both the vagina and the planet.

SUSTAINABLE PRODUCTS

Each time we reuse an item, we reduce its impact on the Earth. In India, the breathable cotton pads are direct descendants of the good old makeshift cotton sarees, which were used by previous generations of women. Modifications have been made to these cloth pads, using sustainable, easy- to-wash and absorbent materials. They also come in attractive designs and prints to enhance the experience.

We should use cotton pads because of the following reasons:

- They are affordable and cost-effective in the long run, as they can last for 3–5 years if they are maintained well.
- They are natural, eco-friendly, skin-friendly and prevent foul smells in intimate areas.
- They support small businesses, as mostly women are involved in making them.

Pre-soaking pads in warm water for at least half an hour before washing releases all the blood, making it easier to remove blood stains. Drying them under the sun naturally sterilizes the pads and prevents any infection due to repeated use.

But these do have some disadvantages, which are as follows:

- Lack of private or toilet space can make it difficult to wash and dry them
- Stigma around menstruation makes one reluctant to dry pads in the open.
- Even the sight of menstrual blood is disagreeable for many.
- Reusing the pads during travel can be cumbersome.

Everyone requires multiple products based on their circumstances. While you might be at ease with cloth pads in the comfort of your home, you might prefer disposable products while travelling. Whenever feasible, consider opting for environment-friendly cloth pads as a gift to Mother Earth.

In contrast, synthetic, disposable sanitary pads dominate market shelves and are widely used, despite the fact that sanitary napkins take an estimated 600 years to break down.[135] Many individuals prefer disposable sanitary pads due to discomfort with inserting a cup or tampon into their vagina. Women often opt for disposable sanitary pads due to their busy schedules, involving significant time spent on work and travel.

Why are they so popular? They are:

- compact and convenient, with no hassle of maintenance.
- suitable travel companions.
- equipped with adhesive strips to keep them in place.
- uncomplicated, as they do not require insertion into the vagina.

Why say 'no' to these pads? Because they are:

- for one-time use only.

[135]Harrison, Megan E., and Nichole Tyson, 'Menstruation: Environmental Impact and Need for Global Health Equity,' *International Journal of Gynecology & Obstetrics*, Vol. 160, No. 2, 2023, 378–382, https://doi.org/10.1002/ijgo.14311.

- not cost-effective.
- ephemeral and finally settle down as landfill waste.
- unsafe, as their extended use can result in the chemicals irritating delicate skin. Moreover, endocrine-disrupting chemicals found in menstrual products can potentially cause cervical cancer.[136,137] Discarded pads may harbour bacteria when exposed to nature.
- artificially scented, and may contain pesticide residues, dioxins and adhesive chemicals, which may cause allergies, rashes, cancer or infections in the reproductive organs.[138]

Philanthropic individuals and activists are raising their voices against such products, rightly advocating for the restriction and gradual elimination of anything that cannot be recycled or composted. Exploring cost-effective alternatives to traditional menstrual products opens doors to sustainable and budget-friendly options. Reusable cloth pads, menstrual cups and period underwear have emerged as eco-conscious alternatives that not only reduce environmental impact but also prove economical in the long run. These choices offer a one-time investment with the potential to last for years, minimizing the monthly expense associated with disposable products. Embracing such alternatives not only benefits the pocket but also contributes to a greener, more sustainable approach to feminine hygiene.

---

[136] Cunningham, Mary, 'Endocrine-disrupting Chemicals Found in Menstrual Products Including Tampons, Pads, and Liners,' *George Mason University*, 15 December 2023, https://www.gmu.edu/news/2023-12/endocrine-disrupting-chemicals-found-menstrual-products-including-tampons-pads-and.

[137] Rachon, Dominik, 'Endocrine Disrupting Chemicals (EDCs) and Female Cancer: Informing the Patients,' *Reviews in Endocrine & Metabolic Disorders*, Vol. 16, No. 4, 2015, 359–364, https://doi.org/10.1007/s11154-016-9332-9.

[138] Upson, Kristen, Jenni A. Shearston, and Marianthi-Anna Kioumourtzoglou, 'Menstrual Products as a Source of Environmental Chemical Exposure: A Review from the Epidemiologic Perspective,' *Current Environmental Health Reports*, Vol. 9, No. 1, 2022, 38–52, https://doi.org/10.1007%2Fs40572-022-00331-1.

Use of Incinerators

With advancements in science, we now have incinerators to support the ecosystem by burning single-use sanitary pads. They reduce pollution to a great degree when they follow eco-friendly guidelines. However, they are not a standalone solution to the pad problem, as they have to be operated in a controlled environment. Therefore, disposable pads should be a security blanket only when no other options are available, rather than a monthly fixture.

Eco-friendly and Disposable

Sanitary pads are in close proximity to our reproductive organs for long periods. Those looking for disposable pads can opt for pads made of greener options available in the market, such as banana fibre, bamboo pulp, wood pulp, bamboo charcoal and hemp.

Advantages

- They are viable, comfortable, earth-friendly, highly absorbent and free from harmful chemicals.
- Their low rate of infections and easy disposal make them the recommended choice of doctors and gynaecologists.
- These pads are classified as biodegradable, with the manufacturers claiming that they decompose within six months of disposal.

Disadvantages

- They are not cost-effective, with genuine ones being highly priced.
- One has to be cautious about brands that claim sustainability and may mislead the public by using synthetic ingredients under the 'eco-friendly' tag.

Embracing eco-consciousness is a commitment we all uphold for the well-being of Mother Earth for healthy evolution and a better tomorrow. The new era is moving towards biodegradable materials, and it is in our best interests to go with the flow.

Tampons

Tampons are small, cylindrical products inserted into the vagina to absorb menstrual blood. Regular tampons were the go-to products before menstrual cups entered the market. These tampons have plastic applicators that take 500 years to decompose, which makes you reconsider using them.

Those comfortable with tampons can opt for eco-friendly ones made with organic cotton. They are attached to reusable applicators with biodegradable packaging. There are also non-applicator tampons that are smaller and more environmentally friendly. These products are all free from pesticides, synthetic materials and bleach, making them safe to use.

Advantages

- Compact, convenient and travel-friendly.
- Highly absorbent, effective and fragrance-free, to prevent allergies.
- Excellent options for sportspersons, as there is no worry of leaks.
- Easy disposal of products due to their compact size.
- Reduces the use of plastic through reusable applicators that can be sterilized.

Disadvantages

- Tampons left within the body for long hours can mess with the PH levels of the vagina, causing irritation and bacterial infections in the vaginal lining.

- High absorbency levels may cause extreme dryness and in rare cases lead to a life-threatening complication called the 'toxic shock syndrome.'
- Cultural beliefs around virginity and rupture of hymen due to insertion discourage tampon use among unmarried girls.
- Increases menstrual symptoms like cramps.
- Takes time and practice for beginners to insert correctly.
- Risk of forgetting to remove them from the body is common and hazardous.

Tampons come in different sizes based on absorbency. They can be:

1. Slender, light ones for beginners and teenagers with a light flow.
2. Regular ones for those with a normal flow.
3. Super-high absorbent ones for women with a heavy flow.

Choosing to opt for a tampon at any age is a personal decision that should be normalized.

Sustainable Underwear

These are innovations of modern life that promote the concept of 'free bleeding' and help one live through menstruation without the hassle of any menstrual products. These undergarments double up as protection pads and come with in-built layers designed to act as moisture barriers. They are reusable, skin and environment-friendly and can hold one to two tampons' worth of flow. Constructed to look and feel like regular underwear, they are available in classic styles, such as high-waist, hip-huggers and even thongs, with different grades of absorption. They are great alternatives for period pads.

Advantages

- Long-lasting.
- Rash-free.
- Clean and dry feel because of their super-absorbent material.
- Anti-odorous, anti-bacterial and easy-to-wash.
- Some products have handy inserts that allow for extra absorption.

Disadvantages

- Highly priced.
- Changing reusable panties can be more challenging than changing reusable pads, especially in public or privacy-restricted washrooms.
- Washing and drying can pose a challenge.
- Not preferred by many as it gives the feeling of wearing a diaper.
- Some manufacturers use synthetic forms of plastic that add to plastic pollution.

Period panties are a great option for those looking for solutions less irritable than tampons and more comfortable than sanitary pads. But despite being promoted as 'life-changers' for women and the ecosystem, these products are mostly relied upon only during lighter flow days.

Menstrual Cups

These are steadily gaining popularity as the most sustainable and ecologically sound option. Made from 100% medical-grade rubber or silicone, they are funnel-shaped and come in different sizes. They can be easily inserted into the vagina to collect blood. Selecting the appropriate cup size relies on factors such as your cervix height, menstrual flow and whether you have given birth vaginally.

Based on available information, manufacturers typically provide two size options: a smaller and a larger one. These sizes may be labelled differently across brands, such as small and large, B and A or models 1 and 2. It is important to note that size variations can exist between brands, and the size designation does not always correlate with the cup's blood-holding capacity.[139]

Advantages

- Last for 8–10 hours without any worry of leakage.
- Available in a choice of colours.
- Safe and non-risky, as long as the cup is used carefully.
- Reusable, environment-friendly and easy to maintain.
- Is expensive but proves to be economical in the long run. With a shelf life of up to 10 years with proper maintenance, menstrual cups have become the most viable option in the market.

Disadvantages

- Dyed silicones can be highly destructive to the environment.
- It may take women some time to feel comfortable inserting the cup.
- Can be messy until mastered to perfection.
- Rare cases of allergy to rubber or latex.
- Choosing the right size to avoid discomfort; getting accustomed to insertions and removals takes time.
- Can cause infections if not sterilized properly.
- Can disrupt the downward flow of the wind or vata, according to alternative therapists.
- Creates irrational fear that insertions might rupture the

[139] West, Mary, 'What to Know About Menstrual Cup Sizing,' *Medical News Today*, Healthline Media, 22 August 2023, https://www.medicalnewstoday.com/articles/menstrual-cup-sizing.

hymen in unmarried girls.

- Those who experience IUDs need to consult a doctor before using them.

Menstrual cups can get easy to use over time. Sterilize your cups by boiling them for 5–10 minutes before every use. Rinsing them thoroughly with non-toxic mild soaps and in lukewarm water after every use can remove any blood residue and keep them hygienic.

CHOOSE THE RIGHT ONE

With so many eco-friendly options available, there are no right or wrong choices; there are only sensible choices.

- Do your research and identify what works best based on your individual needs, comfort, lifestyle, nature of work and preferences.
- Confirm that the pads, tampons and period panties you choose are 100% natural and organic cotton and menstrual cups are 100% silicone.
- Use the ones that best fit your criteria and convenience according to the situation. For example, period panties can be used at home while cups or tampons are best used during physical activities. If one is always on the run and trying to make ends meet, then biodegradable, disposable pads may be the right choice. Those working from home can buy reusable cloth pads.

Be a green warrior by moving away from plastics in your menstrual products as we do not have a Planet B to fall back upon. Look for genuine products from transparent and ethical manufacturers who list their full ingredients. Being a conscious consumer is about choosing the products that are personally suited for your different flows.

The following health apps can also help in planning your life around your menstrual cycle:

1. **Flo:** This app can be your ovulation calendar, period tracker and pregnancy app all rolled into one. Use it to remind and prepare yourself for your next period.
2. **Moon:** This app is a lunar calendar that shows which phase of the Moon you are in.

THE COLOUR SAYS IT ALL

Conversely, knowing the colour of your period blood is as important as choosing the right kind of sustainable products. Your period is governed by your hormonal levels and any imbalance will affect the colour of your bleeding.

The menstrual fluid you see on your pad, tampon or in your menstrual cup is composed of a combination of blood and tissue shed from the uterus lining. The appearance and consistency of the fluid are influenced by the ratio and quantity of blood and tissue, which can vary from person to person and from cycle to cycle. Overall, a healthy menstrual cycle is reflected in the characteristics of the menstrual fluid.

As your menstrual cycle progresses, be mindful of any changes in the colour and consistency of your flow. A possible indication of early pregnancy may be seen in a decrease in the flow accompanied by swollen breasts, nausea or vomiting. Dark red flow may occur at the start or end of your period, as the blood is aged or oxidized and takes longer to exit the uterus. Black discharge, with potential symptoms of pain and clotting, may be present in those with a history of fibroids or severe endometriosis. Grey discharge may signify a bacterial infection, while orange discharge may indicate a mix of menstrual blood and cervical fluid, a sign of possible infection accompanied by itching or odour. Though variations in colour are common and not always concerning, unusual colours such as grey warrant immediate consultation with a healthcare provider.

THE BOTTOM LINE

Have the courage to break the shackles of patriarchy and emerge from the feeling of disgust and shame around menstruation. However, the struggle is far from over. Our menstrual cycles are disrupted because of the emotional environment within, due to genetic conditions, personal traumas and societal conditions. Let us promote this wisdom by openly discussing it, educating others and advocating for menstrual health rights. Together we can create a world where menstruation is celebrated as a natural and essential part of life.

NIMMI'S MANTRA

Take that one conscious step towards going green to honour Mother Earth, and you are inadvertently taking a giant leap towards your health and well-being.

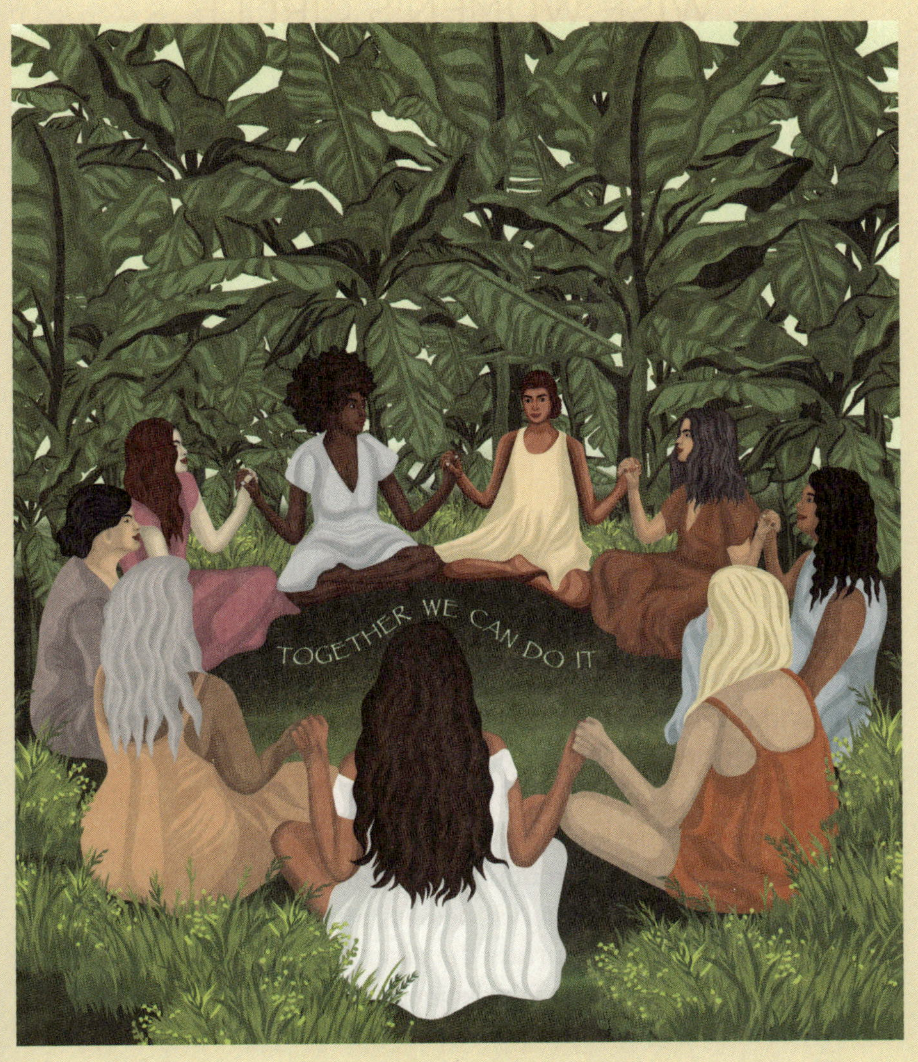
TOGETHER WE CAN DO IT

17

WISE WOMEN'S CIRCLE

'The Circle has healing power.
In the Circle, we are all equal.
When in the Circle, no one is in front of you
No one is behind you.
No one is above you. No one is below you.
The Sacred Circle is designed to create unity.'

—DAVE CHIEF

In the sacred space of a 'wise woman's circle,' every woman finds sanctuary, bound together by love and care. It is a supportive community where women are heard, respected and uplifted with a deep sense of camaraderie. These circles provide more than just support; they offer invaluable guidance, helping women maintain their morale and persevere with grace. By weaving a bond of sisterhood, they support healing and foster feelings of benevolence.

Now, let us not overlook the significance I am trying to convey here. As women, we possess a unique power to give life, to create and to nurture the essence of femininity within ourselves. We are inherently distinct from men, and it is crucial not to underestimate our potential. Authentic feminine energy flourishes best when not overshadowed by masculine energy or stresses of survival, as these can significantly disrupt the delicate balance of our body's bio-rhythm.

In an era dominated by competitiveness and the pervasive influence of masculine energy, women often unconsciously embrace its negative aspects, resulting in unhealthy dynamics such as stress, jealousy and excessive competition. However, being constantly in an aggressive or competitive state can disrupt the innate feminine hormones, leading to distress in reproductive health and overall well-being. To preserve both menstrual and mental health, it is imperative for women to rediscover their essence, find their way to their true feminine selves and cultivate harmony with their hormones.

Consider this chapter not as a directive, but as an invitation to embrace and foster creativity and champion inclusivity. By doing so, we can flourish in a realm of healthy feminine polarity, where balance and well-being are cherished above all else.

THE HISTORY OF CIRCLES

In ancient times, women's gatherings were also known as 'Moon Circles', held chiefly during the waxing and waning periods to harness the Moon's power as a way to manifest feminine energies (as detailed in Chapter 3). Moon Circles enabled women to get insights into the Moon's influence on the human psyche and our ancestors availed it as an antidote to heal and to manifest during various phases of menstrual cycles.

These gatherings began as community rituals aimed at collectively enhancing feminine energy and finding solace during times of struggle. These rituals served as a source of inspiration for the vulnerable and marginalized, providing support to build mental resilience and reclaim control over their lives.

Over time, these circles attracted women from diverse backgrounds, including visionaries, scientists, spiritual seekers and healers, all united for the betterment of the community.

History lauds the role of such women who played a significant part in building iconic role models, whose influence endures even today. Such was the power of women coming together to uplift and empower each other.

The strength of these gatherings also brought a sense of well-being within the community and helped maintain an unbiased balance between genders.

MILLENNIAL WOMEN

You might be wondering why the modern woman needs such women's circles! Why does she require a community and its support amidst her worldly aspirations to ponder over the need to embody femininity in her life? Irrespective of the answer, modern societal expectations directly impact and disrupt the flow of energy, subsequently affecting women's reproductive and emotional health.

Contemporary society has made monetary gain and worldly perfection its chief focus by rewarding people who over-exert their minds and bodies. The pull of victory, success, popularity and self-glory is making women retreat from their inherent feminine traits. This illusion of peripheral attraction is overwhelming and can be challenging for many to handle with grace and calm, without succumbing to negative traits such as ego, jealousy, greed and fear. Women are compelled to disregard their self-care in pursuit of monetary returns and achieving targets and powerful positions with a lack of boundaries. This leaves them discontented with no quality time for meaningful relationships or fulfilling hobbies.

Undoubtedly, women are scaling unprecedented heights with financial success and multiple accolades in their chosen careers, but alas, these achievements are also laced with low tolerance levels and troubling behaviours and attitudes. They are struggling to strike a balance between their goals and well-being, and are unable to handle the pressures of the competitive environment without compromising their health.

In truth, women who lack confidence or exhibit timidity are at risk of mistreatment, not just by men but also by other women. Their reluctance to assert themselves and inability to say no can leave them open to exploitation and manipulation.

Moreover, there are hypersensitive and troubled women battling inner conflicts due to differences with their family and their dear ones. A lack of compassion or a breach of trust can easily turn these inner struggles into emotional turmoil, hindering personal growth and leading to personality disorders, depression and anxiety.

Community alienation is another matter of concern. When society intervenes in a woman's personal choices, the pressure to align with society's values can be stressful and bewildering. A woman is criticized for choosing domestic life and motherhood over a professional one or prioritizing their chosen career path over marriage. These are personal decisions that are solely hers to make, and the biased and opinionated criticisms without proper consideration can cause chaos.

Additionally, beauty standards are often manufactured and manipulated by social media to feed off of the ignorant and to exploit women's insecurities. Modern society makes people believe that only external beauty is worthy of appreciation, even if it is artificial, consisting of heavily filtered images or other superficial enhancements.

It is ironic that women need to be constantly reminded to redirect their focus towards self-care and savour the simple joys of life—pausing, breathing and nourishing their bodies, as they are all essentials for a harmonious life. The value of these practices may only become apparent when faced with illness, mental health challenges, loss of loved ones or mortality itself.

WHY WOMEN'S CIRCLES?

'The circles of women around us
weave invisible nets of love
that carry us when we are weak
and sing with us when we are strong.'

—SARK

Now more than ever, it is crucial to revive women-centric gatherings to harness the power of feminine energy and offer support, regardless of status, religion, colour or caste. The focus isn't on the past or where one comes from but on forging ahead into the future.

Women's circles have the power to weave invisible nets of love among women. They can uplift the weak, applaud the strong and honour the ordinary with no sense of shame. Within these circles women are encouraged to shed their superwoman personas, finding space, clarity and time for self-reflection while channelling their energies towards realistic goals. The circle serves as a constant reminder to cherish and celebrate every role—whether that of a dynamic entrepreneur, devoted mother, efficient fundraiser, creative artist or benevolent giver.

The unwavering support within the circle helps women to amplify their sense of belonging and seek mutual assistance. One woman can provide a sense of community and belonging to another, helping her overcome past bitterness or fear of failure, or merely being a pillar of support to shift focus from resentment by replacing it with compassion.

These circles inspire women to view each other not as competitors or adversaries but as allies. They foster a balance of healthy masculine and feminine energies, offering guidance to discover the true meaning of inner polarities and instilling confidence to coexist with individuals holding diverse views and perspectives.

This shift in energy sets off a ripple effect—a phenomenon where a woman, wounded and healed, touches the soul of another, who in turn extends the healing to others, thereby multiplying the positive vibrations of the circle and increasing the aura of the whole community. Women within these circles are naturally grounded, connected and open to sharing their personal stories without the fear of being judged. It is a space infused with energy needed for women to thrive and nurture compassion for themselves and all other living beings.

Once women feel confident and gain clarity in their thinking, they become exemplars and role models for other women, children and anyone they encounter.

THE INVISIBLE NET OF LOVE

'Behind every strong woman is
a tribe of other strong women who have her back.'

—ANONYMOUS

The philosophy of the women's circle is to empower every woman to progress in both thoughts and actions and become an inspiration for one another. Here are a few precepts that each circle should unconditionally focus on:

- Women in today's digital age are heavily influenced by idealized body images portrayed on social media. Therefore, the primary focus of the circle should be to build awareness around positive body image by changing the perspective on how women look at themselves. By instilling confidence and promoting a sense of security in her own skin, regardless of colour, body type or age, she can find firm footing with ease and also compassionately accommodate others into her fold.

- Within the circle, respect, trust and support are paramount in helping women confront the fear of societal criticism. By providing strength to overcome insecurities without belittling their accomplishments, the women's circle serves as a transformative space for healing emotional wounds stemming from various sources such as parental discrimination, childhood trauma, peer pressures, societal expectations, gender bias and patriarchy. By fostering an environment that encourages women to feel empowered to speak up, share their opinions and inspire those still seeking their own voices, the circle becomes a powerful platform for overcoming challenges and reclaiming individual strength and identity.
- Women's circles highlight the validity of choosing a unique path and pursuing it with passion irrespective of societal norms or expectations.
- Comparison is a huge shackle for women and the circles cautiously dismantle these insecurities by encouraging each woman to celebrate her individuality.
- Women, regardless of their background, are susceptible to feelings of envy, a trait arising from activating the negative side of feminine energy due to lack of self-worth. The circle raises consciousness among women to avoid the evils of engaging in negative self-talk within or outside.
- Within the circle, wise women hold up the mirror of truth, enabling others to witness life's dualities of good and evil objectively. The mirror reflects contradictory emotions, such as hate versus courage, admiration alongside of pessimism, and fear juxtaposed with jealousy. Through this reflection, women gain mental clarity, allowing them to perceive the positive aspects of both masculine and feminine aspects,

thus finding practical solutions to life's challenges. Refer to Chapter 6 to gain deeper insight into these inner dualities.

- Labels unwittingly impose pressure and stress on the mind. In a women's circle, women learn to refrain from labelling themselves as people-pleasers, achievers, timid wallflowers or superwomen and instead, they feel empowered to shift their priorities according to their own needs. She learns not to live with a single tag for the rest of her life.
- Women are encouraged to honour and openly address their menstrual experiences with thoughtfulness and pragmatism. This allows her to openly discuss and share their opinions, breaking the taboos surrounding menstruation.
- Women's circle centred around Moon rituals offer an excellent opportunity to align with the celestial energy, promoting deeper passion and connection with life. These circles provide a sacred space for women from their busy schedules and move towards a more meaningful life.

MOON GATHERINGS

The Moon and the seasons have long demonstrated the synchronicity between women and nature. Therefore, aligning with the phases of the Moon is a wise practice for releasing or attracting energy. Engaging in Moon rituals in wise women's circles can increase their benefits manifold.

The new moon gathering is the time to strengthen and plant the seed of intentions. Focus on what you want to do and where you want to be in life. Come together to meditate collectively, which can help manifest positive change and replace negative thought patterns.

Embrace the use of affirmations such as 'I am authentic,' 'I am confident' or 'I am thriving,' as these have the power to transform manifestations. Speaking these affirmations aloud and in unison creates high-energy vibrations. Continuously revisit these intentions at each gathering to gain a clear perspective on your path forward.

A full moon gathering is an opportunity to open hearts and free yourself from anything that no longer serves you. Release anything that does not resonate with you. It is a great time to overcome negative feelings about the self or others. Shed feelings of jealousy, malicious gossip, bitterness, talking poorly about others' success or the pressure to maintain a flawless appearance with a conscious focus on relevant issues.

Close your eyes and visualize the radiant moonlight illuminating your inner consciousness, purifying and elevating your body, mind and spirit. Collectively working on these rituals can bring about a sense of peace and emotional contentment within the entire community.

MY LEARNINGS

'If you realized how beautiful you are,
you would fall at your own feet.'

—BYRON KATIE

Every stage of a woman's life demands care and attention. Whether she is in her 20s, 30s or 40s, each stage requires a conscious decision to prioritize mental and physical health. Drawing from my own life experiences, here are some essential practices for cultivating a fruitful life and nurturing meaningful relationships:

Follow your vision or dreams: Identify the dreams that truly inspire you, whether it is learning a new skill, establishing a new business or pursuing a hobby.

Imbibe new skills: Expand your knowledge by reading widely, listening to relevant podcasts or learning new art forms or languages regularly.

Focus on communication skills: Master the art of reaching out. It is a skill that helps you face hard conversations. Be an active listener and listen to be heard. 'Choose to respond and not react' should be your emotional quotient mantra when connecting with people. Develop the art of communicating your desires positively, as every word you speak has frequencies to which the law of attraction responds.

Become disciplined: Cultivate good time-management skills by adopting a set routine that includes work, rest and recreation, ensuring a healthy work–life balance.

Maintain a planner: Organize your days, weeks and months effectively through daily journaling, providing clarity and structure to your endeavours.

Accept your limitations: Unrealistic expectations can lead to breakdowns, disrupting the balance of life. Understanding your strengths and weaknesses, along with the aptitude to adapt to change, can help you navigate life's challenges with resilience.

Avoid comparing or competing: Aim to improve yourself rather than considering others as competitors. Progressing in your passion helps you thrive better than competing with others' inherent energies.

Set measurable goals: Establish measurable objectives, such as waking up early, spending time with children, shopping for organic groceries or cooking your own food. Ensure you consider the availability of necessary resources, time and manpower needed to accomplish these goals. As Sid Caesar, actor, comedian and writer, said, 'In between goals is a thing called life, that has to be lived and enjoyed.'

Be fearless: Fear can cloud perceptions and judgements and prevent you from reaching your potential. Build up your courage by gradually stretching and pushing yourself to overcome one fear at a time. Taking that calculated risk can help you move forward.

Take a stand: It is easy to say 'yes' to everything, but over-exhaustion can lead to resentment and fatigue. People-pleasers need to learn to weigh consequences and keep priorities in mind before agreeing to any favour or work.

Do not let mistakes define you: Mistakes are stepping stones that teach you how to approach things differently. Hence, forgive yourself and grow wiser. Never regret trying because setbacks do not define your personality; they only create endless possibilities as tomorrow is another day when you can start over.

Safeguard your finances: Financial independence is important for any woman. Avoid overstretching your budget, as the future is a bag of surprises. Budgeting and financial planning are sustainable skills that lead to stress-free living.

Give yourself options: Focusing solely on one channel can drain your energy or lead to boredom. Have a network of people and meaningful hobbies to energize you and nurture your varied interests in life.

Spend time alone: Be fully present and alive in every moment of life. Observe the changes that each season brings and celebrate daily rituals such as eating, pausing, cooking or gazing at the rising sun, listening to soothing music or nature's sounds. Honour yourself and the body you inhabit. Give yourself the love you deserve by embracing these moments as opportunities for solitary joy and celebration.

Go offline: The digital world isn't reality. Overcome social media addiction by gradually increasing offline time and boosting productivity in all aspects of life. A social media detox also reduces social comparisons and boosts self-esteem.

Take meaningful breaks: Take meaningful breaks to escape the mundane. Even if it is uncomfortable, it ultimately leads to liberation.

Reach out: Stay connected with those who bring value to your life, as they emanate positive energy. A compliment can uplift others and enhance your own emotional state as well. Simultaneously, develop the art of distancing yourself from toxic individuals who consistently drain your energy levels.

Connect with your spirit: Who can appreciate yourself better than you? Be a spiritual seeker and discover what helps you to evolve, as this is the way to nourish your soul. Connect with those enlightened souls who aid in your quest for a deeper understanding of your existence.

Forgive more: Cultivate the habit of forgiving yourself first, then extend forgiveness to all family members whom you feel have wronged you. Absolve any hard feelings you have towards colleagues, neighbours, friends and relatives. Some relationships need reconciliation through healing, others are best left behind with an act of forgiveness. Accept that some situations cannot be changed; instead, focus on shifting your perspective.

Practise gratitude: The universe constantly communicates with us through various signs including pain, loss or obstacles that are guiding us to slow down. Acknowledge every small gesture with gratitude for what you have and what is working in your favour.

Volunteer to make a difference: Dedicate time each week to volunteer for those less fortunate. By contributing to society and your community, you will also enrich your emotions and spirit.

Seek help: Life is not about perfection. It is about enjoying good mental health and leading a healthy life without relying solely on pills. If needed, seek the guidance of a professional therapist. Sometimes, a shift in perspective is all that is needed.

Life can never be perfect for anyone. Use these life lessons to your advantage. Women have been gifted with menstruation by nature for a reason. Be mindful of what each phase of the menstrual cycle offers as the variations in each cycle serve as guiding forces that direct you towards the path of ultimate sublimity.

'Bring in Wintertime with perseverance
for better times to come,
Bring in Spring with innocence
to give shape to all plans and dreams,
Bring in Summertime with exuberance
to enjoy vitality at its peak, and finally
Surrender to the Rainy season with reverence and humility,
for each menstrual phase brings a new perspective to life.'

—ANONYMOUS

THE BOTTOM LINE

Women must overcome a long history of societal shame and embrace the significance of menstrual health. Moreover, chasing superficial goals and seeking external validation has shifted the focus from valuable messages conveyed through the sacred energy centre. These diversions are affecting hormonal health, leading to menstrual discomforts and disrupting the quality of life.

The Circle of Women stands as one of the most powerful forces known to humanity. These are the women who affirm 'Trust your Universe. It has your back.' If you are part of such a circle, embrace it. If you seek one, pursue it. If you find one, then without hesitation, step in and hold on, for it has the power to transform the fabric of your being. You will be changed—for good, better and the best!

NIMMI'S MANTRA

What goes around, comes around. Be the change, heal yourself and help heal others. Become a wise woman, lead women's circles and set examples for others to follow.

ACKNOWLEDGEMENTS

First and foremost, I would like to thank Deepa Venkatesh, creative writer and editor, whose meticulous editing of the manuscript was both prompt and gracious. Her dedication, expertise and unwavering support were invaluable in refining the content and shaping the book into its polished form.

I also acknowledge Dr Aruna Sahadev, a consultant obstetrician, gynaecologist and infertility specialist, whose profound insights into women's health have significantly enhanced the depth and credibility of this book. I am immensely grateful for your expert guidance, which played a pivotal role in bringing this important project to fruition.

Special thanks to Dr Sanmathi P Rao, an ayurvedic consultant, for her contributions to this book. Her commitment to holistic well-being has added a unique perspective to the content, enriching it with insights from the realm of Ayurveda.

Menstruation: Moon, Men and More is the culmination of years of research and data collected from various sources, as well as interactions with numerous individuals and deep introspection. I owe my sincere gratitude to everyone who supported me in this endeavour, including my family and close friends as well as the team at Rupa Publications.

Finally, I wish to express my appreciation to fellow authors, bloggers and illustrators on Pinterest whose insightful blog posts, thought-provoking articles, engaging narratives and creative illustrations served as guiding lights for this book. Your efforts have been instrumental in shaping my own approach to writing, and I aim to honour them by producing a book that not only reflects the wisdom of previous generations of women but also contributes meaningfully to the ongoing conversation. My sincere apologies if I inadvertently missed acknowledging anyone who has contributed to my journey.